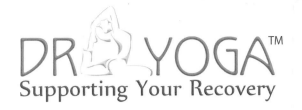

DR YOGA™
Supporting Your Recovery

CW00569805

YOGA

FOR **BREAST CANCER SURVIVORS** AND **PATIENTS**

BY **DR JIMMY KWOK** PHD, RYT200

Copyright © Jimmy Kwok, 2017
Published by I_AM Self-Publishing, 2017.

The right of Jimmy Kwok to be identified as the Author of the Work has been asserted by him in accordance with the Copyright, Designs and Patents Act 1988.

All rights reserved.

ISBN 978-1-911079-45-3

This book is sold subject to the condition it shall not, by way of trade or otherwise, be circulated in any form or by any means, electronic or otherwise without the publisher's prior consent.

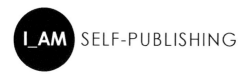

🐦 iamselfpub
www.iamselfpublishing.com

Yoga for Breast Cancer Patients and Survivors

The Practice Manual

- *With guided sequences of three levels of difficulties, helping you to progress through your journey into your recovery*
- *Suitable as a tool for a home-based practice*

Medical information provided by Dr Yoga must be considered as an educational service only. This book is not designed to replace a doctor's independent judgement about the appropriateness or risks of a procedure or therapy for a given patient. Dr Yoga aims to provide you with information to make your own decisions to support your recovery.

The information provided in this book are believed to be accurate and sound at the time of writing and readers who fail to consult appropriate medical advice from appropriate health authorities assume the risk of any injuries, accidents or death. The author, editors and publishers are not responsible for errors and disclaim any liabilities or loss in connection with the exercise and advice herein.

About Dr Yoga

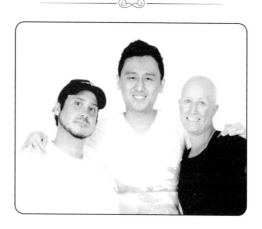

Dr Yoga® was founded by Dr Jimmy Kwok in 2016 to promote the benefits that yoga could bring for cancer patients and recovering survivors. Jimmy gained his MA in Natural Sciences from Emmanuel College, University of Cambridge and his doctorate degree in Clinical Oncology (Breast Cancer) at Imperial College, London. Jimmy has also interned at Harvard Medical School, Boston, USA and the Oncology Department at Great Ormond Street Hospital, London. He has practised Ashtanga yoga for over a decade and he is also a registered Yoga Alliance UK RYT200 yoga instructor. Furthermore, he has developed extensive experience in promoting and teaching yoga classes at Maggie's Cancer Centre, West London, within the NHS Charing Cross Hospital Campus.

He has recognised that the psychological, emotional and physical support for cancer patients is often overlooked, and has developed a series of home-based materials in supporting the recovery for cancer patients and survivors.

Visit Dr Yoga's website at **www.dryoga.co.uk** for further information.

Foreword

Yoga (a Sanskrit word) is a commonly-known generic term for physical, mental, and spiritual disciplines, which originated in ancient India. The literal meaning is translated as "yoke" and it is generally interpreted as a practice or path that can lead to the perfection of "stillness", both physically and mentally. Specifically, yoga belongs to one of the six ("orthodox") schools of Hindu philosophy, based on the *Yoga Sūtras of Patañjali*. Various traditions of yoga can also be found in Hinduism, Buddhism, Jainism and Sikhism. Someone who follows the yogic practices is often called a *Yogi* (male) or *Yogini* (female).

In essence, yoga involves the practice of physical *asanas* (postures) and *pranayama* (breath control) to create *pratyahara* (sense withdrawal), which increases the mental focus, or known as *dharana* (concentration) of the *yogi* or *yogini*. The increased concentration forms the foundation for *dhyana* (meditation) in achieving *Samadhi* (a state of inner joy/peace) during the practice. By adopting yoga practices, it assists *yogi* or *yogini* in the cultivation of *niyama* (self-awareness) in daily living, thus encouraging the adoption of *yama* (ethical principles) in daily lives.

Swami Vivekananda was the first Hindu monk that brought yoga to the West in the late 19th century. He was the first Hindu teacher to actively advocate and disseminate yoga teachings to Western audiences by touring Europe and the United States in the 1890s. Overcoming initial sceptical receptions, it took nearly another century before yoga finally gained mainstream acceptance as a form of legitimate health exercise in the Western world in the second half of the 20th century. The evolution of Hatha yoga in the Western world has also witnessed a loss of the spiritual or meditation practices found in traditional ancient yoga practices, where the mental, psychological and spiritual benefits to yoga practitioners are not harnessed. In recent years, newer schools of yoga like Yin yoga and Insight yoga are gaining prominence to revive these missing elements, making yoga more than just a form of exercise.

With Western scientific rigour, in the past decade, there has been an explosion of clinical and scientific studies performed to validate the effectiveness of yoga as a complementary, therapeutic intervention for cancer. Several studies have been shown to improve musculo–skeletal and mental health of cancer patients. Cancer survivors who also engage in regular yoga practice also show an increase in brain (GABA) Gamma-aminobutyric levels, improving mood and anxiety more than some other metabolically-matched exercises, such as walking. The emergence of recent studies investigating yoga as a complementary intervention for cancer patients by very prominent scientific researchers, including the MD Anderson Cancer Centre in USA, has given clinical support to the use of yoga as part of an integrative modality in treating cancer patients and cancer survivors. They have shown that yoga reduces the levels of stress hormone cortisol in breast cancer patients, which is correlated with a better treatment prognosis outcome. Other Mindfulness Based Stress Reduction (MBSR) programmes, including yoga as a mind-body technique, have also demonstrated yoga's effectiveness in alleviating the most common effects of radiotherapy and chemotherapy, including depression, stress, mood swings, insomnia, pain, and fatigue and anxiety. All of this translates into a better quality of life for recovering cancer patients and survivors.

This book is dedicated to everyone who has been affected by cancer, and that they can find both solaces and strength from their yoga practice.

Best Wishes,

Jimmy Kwok

Acknowledgements

First and foremost, I would like the express my sincere gratitude to all the past yoga gurus for their wisdom and millennia of dedication in passing down the rich tradition of yoga beings to benefit countless individuals in their lifetime. I have also been humbled and privileged to have studied under the guidance of several great yoga teachers, including Ryan Spielman, Phillipa Gendall, Sarai Harvey Smith and Elinore Burke.

I would also like to thank Jo Taylor, breast cancer patient and survivor, and founder of ABCdiagnosis, for her participation in the photo shoot and my admiration for her bravery and dedication to help other women recovering from breast cancer. Also, I would like to thank Scott Danaeza, who has helped to take the beautiful photographs for this book, without which this project wouldn't have happened.

Last but not least, I would also like to thank my family for their love and continued support.

Author Biography

Jimmy is currently working for a private hospital group based in Harley Street, London, UK as the Head of Oncology Service Line. In his role, he is responsible for the management and development of the cancer services across the network of UK facilities. He has gained his MA in Natural Sciences from Emmanuel College, University of Cambridge, and his PhD in Clinical Oncology at Imperial College, London.

Jimmy has also interned at other prominent institutions, including the Harvard Medical School, Boston USA and the Institute of Child Health and Great Ormond Street Hospital, London. Furthermore, Jimmy is an experienced and registered RYT-200 Yoga Alliance. He has practiced Ashtanga yoga for over a decade and he still frequently visits India for further yoga and meditation training. Throughout the years, Jimmy has also regularly worked closely and taught at Maggie's London Cancer Centre, adjacent to NHS Charing Cross Hospital, to promote the use of yoga in recovering cancer patients and survivors.

What is Cancer?

Cancer is essentially a form of diseases, which are characterised by an uncontrolled cell growth where tumour cells develop in a series of stages, which may or may not become malignant and metastatic. Metastatic essentially means that cancer cells migrate from their site of origin and anchor themselves into secondary sites.

Tumour development proceeds via a process that is analogous to Darwinian evolution, where a succession of genetic mutations, which confer them an advantage, lead to progressive conversion of normal cells into cancer cells. There are generally six hallmark traits of cancer cell – they have acquired self-sufficiency in growth, signalling biochemical pathways, insensitivity to anti-growth signals, evading mechanisms of regulated cell death, limitless replicative potential, ability to undergo angiogenesis (formation of network of blood vessels), and tissue invasion or metastatic capabilities [1].

Cancer can happen in most parts of the human body, including the most common ones such breast, prostate, lung, kidney, liver, pancreas, brain, and the head and neck.

What is Yoga?

Yoga, in its simplest terms, is a form of physical exercises incorporating mindfulness practices, which assists the practitioner in the "control of thought waves in the mind".

Yoga is an ancient practice, having its roots dated back 2,500 years ago in India, where it came from. One of the most famous Hindu yoga sages and gurus, Patajali, complied the Yoga Sutras, which expounded the theories of yoga practice [2].

The fundamental difference between yoga as a form therapy is it encompasses both the physical and psychological wellbeing for cancer patients and survivors. The practice of physical yoga postures could help improve stamina, core strength and flexibility of muscles, whilst the practice of yoga breathing and mindfulness could help to relieve mental fatigue and depression.

Yoga encourages practitioners to develop an inner awareness of focusing on the breathing, which can help in the cessation of some of the most repetitive, psychologically self-defeating thoughts that one may find themselves encountering whilst undergoing active treatment or transitioning into life beyond cancer. You can then learn to extinguish and become less attached to negative thoughts, and start living your full potential, enjoying what life has to offer.

The table below summarises the key differences between yoga and other physical forms of exercises, and why, in my opinion, yoga could be much more suitable therapy for cancer patients and survivors during or post-surgical operations, chemotherapy and radiotherapy treatment, where the emphasis should be on rejuvenation and restoration of the body, aiding its recovery.

Yoga therapy	Physical exercises
Yoga has been clinically proven to reduce cortisol (stress hormone), which is correlated with better cancer prognosis in patients undergoing cancer treatment [3].	Physical exercises increase adrenaline [4] and high-intensity exercise provokes increases in circulating cortisol levels [5].
Yoga therapy tends to put emphasis on slower movements with longer-held physical postures, which encourages elongation of muscles, and therefore inducing relaxation [6].	Active physical exercises encourage a build-up of lactic acid in muscle fibre, which can cause physical fatigue [7].
Yoga can help in the development of concentration and mindfulness, translating into tangible benefits outside of the yoga mat [8] [9].	Physical exercises tend to be goal-orientated and encourages agenda-driven exercises, which can often inflate egoistic ambitions, not necessarily inducing the right frame of mind for rehabilitation [10].
Yoga stretching forces blood through the valves in the veins, and inversion postures can relax the heart muscles by encouraging blood flow back to the heart. It has also been shown to decrease heart rate variability [11].	Excessive endurance exercises could put significant stress on the heart muscles, resulting in adverse cardiovascular effects [12].

Clinical proven benefits of yoga for cancer patients & survivors

A review of the benefits that yoga might bring to cancer patients and survivors were conducted by CRUK in March 2010, where the scientific rigour of 10 clinical trials performed to date was examined in greater detail [13]. A majority of the clinical trial participants were breast cancer patients. Reported clinical benefits included reduced levels of anxiety, depression, fatigue and stress, improving quality of sleep, mood and spiritual well-being. The assessment was that, on balance, yoga may improve the psychological well-being in cancer recovery for some breast cancer patients, based on these studies, but weak study designs and a low number of participants in some studies prevented a firmer conclusion from being drawn.

However, a recent landmark clinical study has allowed researchers to back up the data from smaller trials and other countless anecdotal evidence of how yoga has been found to benefit cancer patients. Professor Lorenzo Cohen, Director of the Integrative Medicine Program at The University of Texas, MD Anderson Cancer Centre, has performed a clinical study, and the results have suggested that yoga can benefit breast cancer patients under radiotherapy [14]. The study recruited 163 women with stage 0 – 3 breast cancer, lasting over a six-month period. They underwent six weeks of radiotherapy and were randomly assigned into three groups, which received different add-on instructions apart from their standard course of radiotherapy. Group 1 received three hourly yoga sessions per week; Group 2 received three hourly simple stretching exercise regimes per week; Group 3 acted as a control group, who received neither yoga nor stretching regimes. The most significant finding here is that women who practised yoga registered the sharpest fall in a stress hormone – cortisol (hydrocortisone). Cortisol is normally produced by the adrenal gland in response to stress. This is of particular importance because "blunted circadian cortisol rhythm" – a high level of blood cortisol levels in the body – have been linked to worse outcomes in breast cancer. Unsurprisingly, women who practised yoga also reported qualitatively that they have better general health, physical functioning and psychological well-being.

Professor Cohen cited that "Teaching patients a mind-body technique like yoga as a coping skill can make the transition less difficult." What is more important is that the National Cancer Institute in the USA has awarded the largest grant to date for the study of yoga in cancer to Professor Cohen's team, to conduct a proper Phase III clinical trial for breast cancer patients, to determine the scientific mechanism of how yoga can effect a better biological outcome post-radiotherapy treatments. They are also going to assess the cost efficiencies of implementing yoga programmes in hospitals. To date, this is the only known clinical trial going to be performed to address **how** yoga can benefit breast cancer patients.

There have also been reported benefits for lung cancer, prostate cancer and other cancer types, which I have documented in the following table. By no means is this a comprehensive list, but it highlights the most important and recent ones. References are provided, should readers want to find out more on these independent clinical research studies.

Patient Group	Key research findings
Breast cancer survivors	A randomised, controlled three-month trial was conducted with two post-treatment assessments of 200 breast cancer survivors. Yoga reduces both fatigue and inflammation in breast cancer survivors [15].
Breast cancer survivors	A randomised, controlled three-month trial showed that restorative Iyengar yoga intervention reduced inflammation-related gene expression in breast cancer survivors with persistent fatigue [16].
Early stage breast cancer Patients	A randomised, controlled trial of early breast cancer patients. Yoga showed that it assisted in improving quality of life [17].
Prostate cancer patients	68 prostate cancer patients underwent yoga intervention whilst undergoing radiotherapy treatments. Preliminary results have shown improvement in sexual health function and reduction in fatigue. Prostate cancer patients have also reported a better improvement of quality of life [18].
Non-small cell lung cancer patients	4-week intervention period, 9 patients participated in a weekly 45-minute hatha yoga practice and encouragingly reported that patients experienced a reported moderate decrease in symptoms of dyspnoea [19].
Gynaecologic and breast cancer patients	A self-administered questionnaire was sent to 247 potentially eligible women with breast or gynaecological cancer. Patients showed that yoga/meditation helped lymphoedema management [20].
Ovarian and breast cancer Patients	51 cancer patients enrolled in this study and participated in 10-weekly, 75-minute restorative yoga sessions that combined physical postures, breathing, and deep relaxation. Participants reported significant improvements of reduction in depression and anxiety, whilst seeing an overall improvement of the quality of life [21].
Cancer survivors	410 survivors participated in this study and yoga participants demonstrated greater improvements in global sleep quality [22].

Practical checklist before you begin your yoga practice

If you have never practiced yoga before, it can seem daunting to begin your first exercise. I would recommend you develop a regular practice to gain the maximum benefit. What "regular" means varies from person to person, dependent on the status of their active treatment and their general state of health. Do not feel pressurised into doing more than you can and always listen to your body practice with full mindfulness to avoid injuries. I would also recommend that you speak with your physician prior to beginning a yoga programme, in particular, if you are receiving on-going medical treatment for cancer.

Yoga mat	The most important prop is probably a decent quality yoga mat. I would recommend a longer type of mat (over 180 cm) and 10 mm in thickness, which can provide better comfort when practising yoga.
Yoga attire	Loose, comfortable clothing is essential.
Yoga props	There are certain props, including yoga bricks, yoga belts and yoga eye bags, which you may find useful to assist in certain asana practice.
Yoga music	Sometimes, yoga music with yoga chants/sounds of nature can help you to focus your attention on your practice if you are struggling with concentration or holding postures for the ideal duration.
Incense	Sometimes, incense is useful to again, help improve mood or concentration of focus during the yoga practice.
Time of practice	It is advisable not to practise yoga immediately after food. I would recommend three hours of interval between a large meal and yoga practice. Morning is the best time to begin a yoga practice, with a fresh mind and empty stomach, which is the most inductive to a yoga practice session.
Location of practice	It is advisable to practise in a quiet, warm, indoor environment. It can be difficult to focus if practising outdoor.

Breath and Gaze

It would also be important to introduce two basic concepts – breath and gaze – when you are moving through the yoga practice.

It is important to pay attention to your breathing – during both inhalation and exhalation that you maintain a long, smooth breath. Shallow, rapid breathing can create additional anxiety and tension in your body. Just notice your breath coming and going; you will notice that your mind will wander with many thoughts. They may come in the form of "When is my next chemo appointment?", "Have I done my laundry?", "What should I have for lunch?" – lots of noise and chatter. Just learn to acknowledge the thoughts but do not get engaged in them. Bring your attention back to your breathing. This form of yoga practice is adopted from the Buddhist meditation practice called *vipassanna* meditation – which essentially encourages the cultivation of mindfulness. It has numerous physiological benefits and several modern-day practitioners in Psychological Cognitive Behaviour Therapy have derived their models based on mindfulness practices developed over 2,500 years ago.

The other important aspect of yoga practice is your gaze, i.e. where you rest your focus/attention. This is called *drishti* in Sanskrit. By focusing your physical gaze onto an area, you reduce potential distractions, and this helps to quieten your mind by encouraging your consciousness to move inwards. Practising both *drishti* and breathing during your yoga practice can encourage quietening of the mind, and hopefully will result in a sense of peace and calm. There are usually eight *drishti*, which are listed below.

1. *Nasagrai* – top of the nose

2. *Ajna chakra* – between the eyebrows – third eye

3. *Nabi chakra* – navel

4. *Hastagrai* – hand

5. *Padhayoragrai* – toes

6. *Parsva drishti* – far right/far left

7. *Angustha Ma Dyai* – thumbs

8. *Urdhva drishiti* – upwards/ up to the sky

If it is too difficult to practice both breathing and *drishti* in the beginning, you can you always leave these "optional" practices out whilst you focus on the physical postures. Take it at your own pace, and your practice will grow and develop in time.

"Do not lose yourself in the past. Do not lose yourself in the future. Do not get caught in your anger, worries, or fears. Come back to the present moment, and touch life deeply. This is mindfulness."
- Venerable Thich Nhat Hanh, The Heart of the Buddha's Teaching: Transforming Suffering into Peace, Joy, and Liberation

Guided Yoga Sequence For Cancer Patients

Gentle healing yoga flow sequence

The gentle healing yoga flow sequence is specifically designed for cancer patients recovering from surgery or undergoing active treatments like radiotherapy and chemotherapy. The sequence is designed for those who want to alleviate the common side effects of these treatments, including fatigue, insomnia, muscular pain, anxiety and depression.

You should never experience pain in your bones/joints or difficulty in breathing in any of the yoga postures. If you do, back out of the posture and do not go so deep into them. Listen to your body.

The gentle healing yoga flow sequence will take approximately 60 minutes to complete. One is encouraged to follow the order of the sequence to gain the maximum benefits from the practice.

Gentle Healing Yoga Flow Sequence Chart

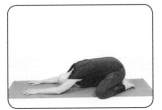

Wide knee child's pose

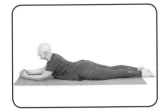

Gentle sphinx

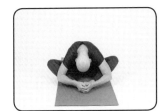

Butterfly

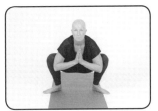

Wide knee squat

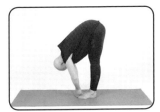

Standing forward bend

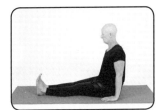

Staff pose

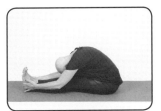

Seated forward bend

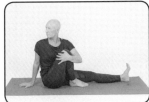

Seated twist

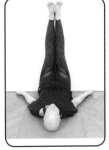

Supported
shoulder stand

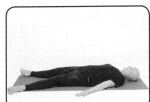

Savasana

Wide Knee Child's Pose

a. Starting with a kneeling position on the floor, knees and feet together, sit on the back of your soles. If you feel pain or discomfort on your knees, come out of the posture and reset, placing a blanket or towel between the thighs and calves.

b. Inhale and bring both knees wide apart, as far as they will go (A).

c. Exhale, reaching forwards with your fingers and rest your forehead onto the floor. Keep both hands straight in front of you and relax completely onto the floor (B). If you head doesn't reach the floor, you can use a bolster for support by placing it in front of your forehead.

d. *Nasagrai drishti* – gazing towards your nose

e. Breathe deeply. Inhale and exhale for 20 breaths.

f. Using your arms for support, gently push yourself up to an upright position

Comments: The wide knee child's pose is a very healing posture and stretches the spine. The gentle compression of the stomach and chest encourages circulation and promotes healing in those areas of the body. Bringing the knees wide apart also stretches and relieves the inner thigh and inner groin muscles. In addition, this pose encourages flow of lymphatic fluid and reduces swelling in the neck, head and limbs for those suffering from lymphedema.

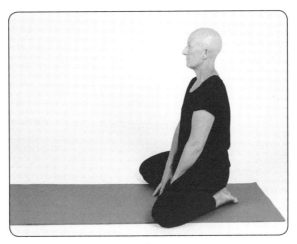

A

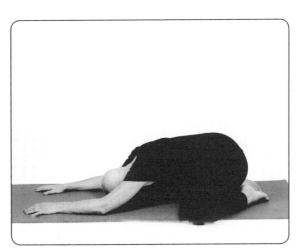

B

Gentle Sphinx

a. Inhale and lie down on the floor, feet flat and resting your chest on the floor with your hands lying next to you.

b. Exhale and gently bring your hands forwards and interlock your fingers together, forming a triangular base for support.

c. Inhale and gently slide your chest/ribs upwards for a gentle backbend, keeping your shoulders relaxed. If this is too intense for you, you can lower your chest and remain closer to the floor.

d. *Nasagrai drishiti* – gazing towards the top of your nose

e. Breathe deeply. Inhale and exhale for 20 breaths.

f. On your last exhale, gently slide your elbows to the side. Turn your head to the right hand side and rest on the floor for 10 breaths. Completely relaxing and letting the weight of the floor support your weight.

g. Inhale, interlocking your fingers together forming a triangular base for support and gently slide your chest/ribs upwards to your comfortable edge.

h. Nasagrai drishiti – gazing towards the top of your nose.

i. Breathe deeply. Inhale and exhale for another 20 breaths.

j. On your last exhale, gently slide your elbows to the side. Turn your head to the left-hand side and rest on the floor for 10 breaths, completely relaxing and letting the weight of the floor support your weight.

Comments: The gentle sphinx posture provides a subtle backbend at the sacral-lumbar arch and helps tone the spine. This posture is particular helpful for those who have undergone breast surgeries, and the gentle indirect chest opening motion helps promote blood circulation to the scar tissue areas, promoting healing.

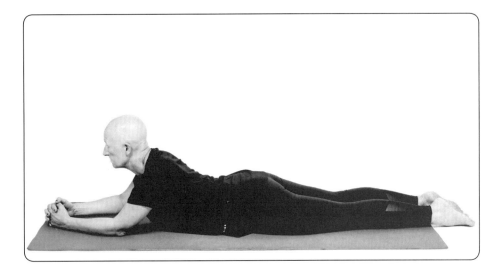

You cannot always control what goes on outside.
But you can always control what goes on inside."
- Wayne Dyer

Butterfly

a. From a lying down position, use your hands to push yourself upwards and transition into a simple cross-legged posture.
b. Inhale, and bring the soles of your together and slide them gently away from you into a "kite" shape.
c. Exhale, gently curling your spine and rolling forwards, bringing the crown of head towards your feet, wrapping your hands around your feet (A). For extra comfort, you can rest your forehead on a pillow or bolster for support (B). If you find it difficult sitting on the floor without support, you can also choose to sit on a block, tilting your pelvis forwards, which can help with bending forwards.
d. *Nasagrai drishti* – gaze towards the top of the nose.
e. Breathe deeply. Inhale and exhale for 20 breaths.
f. On your last inhale, use your hands to push yourself up into an upright position.
g. Exhale and straighten your feet out, leaning back on your hands to release tension in your hips and spine.

Comments: The butterfly posture provides a gentle counter-pose to the sphinx posture. This posture allows for an easy stretch to the lower back, without the need of very open hamstrings. There will also be a stretching sensation along the outer thighs and lower back area. If at any point, pressure or stretch becomes too intense, just ease off the forward bend and do not bend so far forwards.

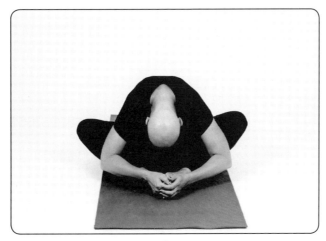

A

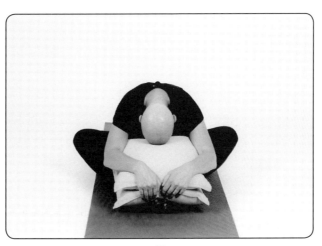

B

Wide Knee Squat

a. Inhale and transition from the last posture into a standing upright position, standing hip-width apart

b. Exhale, squat down slowly, and bring your arms in front of you, both hands resting onto the floor. If your hips are very far off the floor, use the wall for support and squat as far down as you can and stay in the posture (A). If possible, you can also tiptoe and keep your heels slightly above the floor (B).

c. If there isn't too much strain on the knees/feet, you can inhale and come into the full posture by bringing your elbows in towards your inner thighs and holding your hands in a prayer position (C).

d. Exhale, and push your elbows gentle into your inner thighs to open your hips and shoulders further. Avoid collapsing your chest.

e. *Nasagrai drishti* – gaze towards the top of the nose.

f. Breathe deeply. Inhale and exhale for 20 breaths.

g. On your last exhale, gently release your hands and bring them in front of you.

h. Inhale and, with the support of your arms, come all the way up to standing.

Comments: The wide knee squat provides a deep opening to your hips, whilst strengthening your ankle and thigh muscles. It also releases tension on the lower back and provides relief for lower back pain due to inertia or strain. If knees hurt when you come down into a squat, just remain standing and use the wall for support to come as far down as you can. By pressing your elbows against your inner thighs, it also helps relieve tension around the shoulder area, again particular beneficial for those who have undergone a reconstruction surgery.

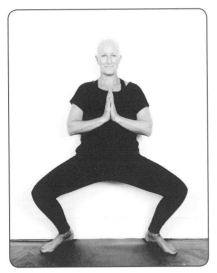

A

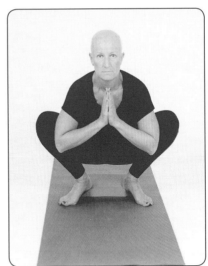

B

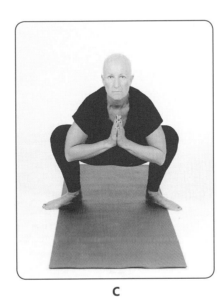

C

Standing Forward Bend

a. Inhale, standing hip-width apart.
b. Exhale. Place your hands onto the waist.
c. Inhale. Lift your chest and tilt your head back gently, gazing towards the sky.
d. Exhale, keeping your legs straight and fold forward, maintaining the length in your spine and bringing your hands just below your knee cap (A), your shin (B), or wrap the first two fingers around your big toe (C), dependent on the flexibility of your hamstring. Let the weight of your head go.
e. *Nasagrai drishti* – gaze towards the top of the nose
f. Breathe deeply. Inhale and exhale for 20 breaths.
g. On your last inhale, gently bring both hands onto your waist.
h. Exhale, look up and gaze forwards.
i. Inhale, gently bringing your back up to an upright position with a straight spine and hands into a prayer position.
j. Exhale, releasing both hands to the side.

Comments: The standing forward bend is a great posture to release tensions in the hamstrings, and tilt the upper pelvis forwards gently to help straighten the spine, providing extra relief on tension around the lower back area. It is important to relax your shoulders in the posture and let the weight on the head hang and align with gravity. If you feel dizzy when coming straight back up, come into the child's pose and rest for a few minutes before moving onto the next posture. Standing forward bend also helps encourage the flow of lymphatic fluid and helps reduce swelling In addition, this pose aims to reducing the swelling in the head and neck areas

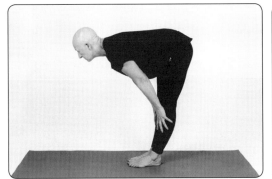

A

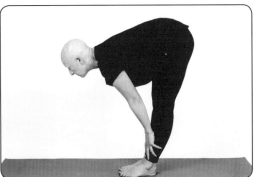

B

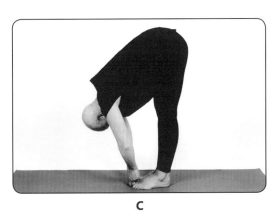

C

Staff Pose

a. From standing, come down to sitting with both legs straight in front you.
b. Inhaling, pressing both hands aligned with your hips onto the floor, chest open and palms flat on the floor (A). If you experience tightness in your lower back and find it hard to keep your spine straight, bend your knees (B) or support the bent knees with extra cushions (C).
c. Exhale, chin down. Keep your legs active and engage your quadriceps. Keep your spine tall and your arms straight.
d. *Nasagrai drishti* – gaze towards the top of the nose and stay here for 10 breaths.
e. Inhale, chin up, and relax your shoulders.

Comments: If your legs are straight, keep the back of the knees pressing down and your heels away to create length in the legs. Whichever variation you choose, remember to keep the shoulder relaxed and keep your chest open in this posture.

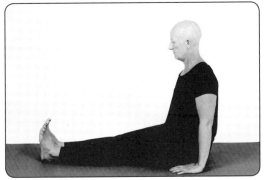

A

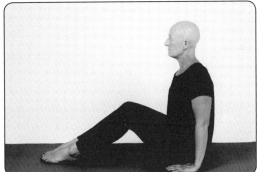

B

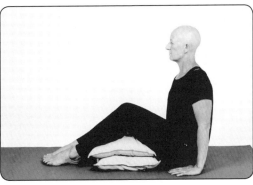

C

Seated Forward Bend

a. From staff pose, inhale and bring both hands up to the sky. Keep your spine straight and shoulders relaxed.

b. *Urdhva drishiti* – gaze towards the sky.

c. Breathing deeply here, hold for five breaths.

d. On your last exhale, keeping both arms straight and your spine straight, forward bend, reaching as far as your hands can reach. Rest your hands on the shin (A) or wrap both hands outside of your feet (B). If your hamstrings are tight, you can also bend forwards with bent knees (C) or with extra support of the cushions (D) and rest your forehead on your thighs.

e. *Padhayoragrai drishti* – gaze towards your toes. Keep your shoulders relaxed.

f. Breathing deeply here. Hold here for 10 breaths.

g. On your last inhale, come back up to a straight spine.

h. Exhale, coming back to a staff pose and rest both hands on the floor next to your waist.

Comments: If you feel discomfort or pain in your lower back, bend your knees and come out of the posture slowly. You should also keep your spine long and shoulders relaxed in the posture, do not pull yourself into the forward bend, as it will only serve to tighten the shoulders more. In addition, this pose encourages flow of lymphatic fluid and reduces swelling in the head and neck area for those suffering from lymphedema.

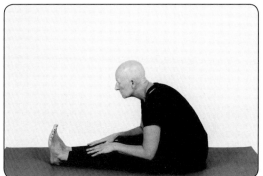

A

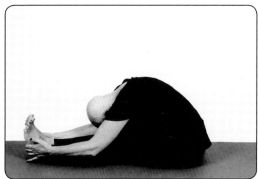

B

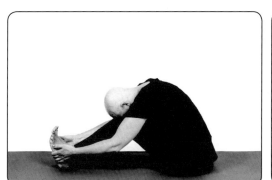

C

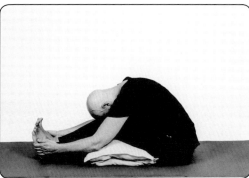

D

Seated Twist

a. From a staff pose, inhale and bend the right leg and place the heel about hip-width apart. Place your right hand on the floor behind you.

b. Exhale, twist and rotate from the lower spine. Hold the right knee with your left hand (A).

c. Inhale, lengthen spine and turn gaze over the right shoulder.

d. *Parsva drishti* – gaze towards the back.

e. Stay here for five deep breaths.

f. Inhale, keeping the spine straight, and rotate and turn your body to the front

g. Exhale; release your hands and straighten both legs.

h. Inhale; place your left hand on floor behind you.

i. Exhale, twist and rotate from the lower spine. Hold the left knee with your right hand (B).

j. Inhale, lengthen spine and turn gaze over the left shoulder.

k. *Parsva drishti* – gaze towards the back.

l. Stay here for another five deep breaths.

m. Inhale, keeping your spine straight, and rotate and turn your body to the front.

n. Exhale; release your hands and straighten both legs.

Comments: This posture is especially helpful for those who have undergone a reconstruction surgery, where the shoulders/chest area can be very tight. If you find that your lower back hunches too much in this posture and it is preventing you from twisting to the side, sit on a yoga block to add some height and help straighten the spine. It also helps stretch and loosen the spine, toning and conditioning the nerves along the spinal cord. It can also help to relieve neck pain and mild forms of sciatica.

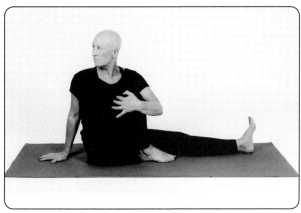

A

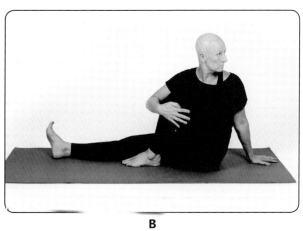

B

Supported Shoulder Stand

a. Bring your hips as close to a wall as much as possible.
b. Lie down on the floor, resting your back and shoulders onto the floor.
c. Inhale, straightening both legs up to the sky with the support of the wall and relaxing both hands to side of the floor, palms up, facing the sky (A).
d. *Urdhva drishiti* – gaze upwards to the sky.
e. Keep breathing deeply. Hold here for five to ten minutes. If you start experiencing pins and needles in your feet during inversions, you can bend your knees slightly (B).
f. On your last exhale, roll over onto your right shoulder and rest there for five breaths.
g. Inhale; with the support of your right hand, push yourself up to a seated position.

Comments: If you feel discomfort or pain in the neck, back off and come out of the posture. Ensure weight of your body is distributed evenly across the shoulders and your back in this posture. Sometimes, shoulder stands are called the Queen of all yoga postures, and many benefits have been associated with this posture, including decreasing varicose veins, reducing your heart rate, regulating hormone production, massaging the thyroid glands and strengthening of the immune system. This is particularly helpful in the case of swollen feet where the flow of the lymphatic fluid accumulated in the feet will move towards the body.

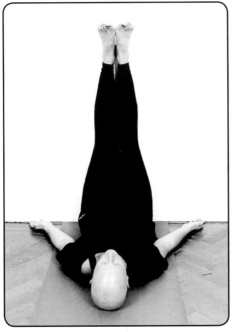

A

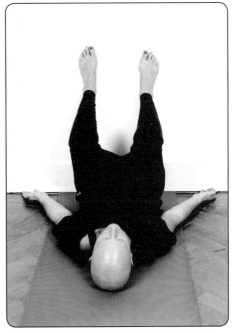

B

Final Relaxation – Savasana

a. From a seated position, inhale and bring your legs out slightly wider than hip-width apart.
b. Exhale, and with the support of your elbow, come to lie down on your back.
c. Inhale; bring your hands away from your waist and open your palms up, facing the sky.
d. Exhale and close your eyes.
e. Breathe normally here and totally relax your body. Release any unwanted tension you may have.
f. Stay here for 10 – 15 minutes and let your body absorb the impact of your practice

Comments: In this final posture, let go of any tension of your body and let it sink into the ground fully, which is supporting your weight. Focus on your breath here and observe the quality of your breath, without judgement. Try to find a place of stillness in your mind and enjoy the tranquillity.

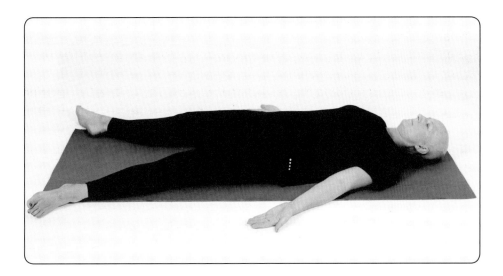

"The Fruits of Yoga Mature With Patience And Care"
- David Swenson, Ashtanga Yoga Master

Rejuvenating Yoga Flow Sequence

The rejuvenating yoga flow sequence is specifically designed for cancer patients who have completed all on-going medical treatments and have moved onto "survivorship" mode. The sequence is also suitable for those who want to start rebuilding their strength and practice through a physically stronger, yet grounded yoga practice.

You should never experience pain in your bones/joints or difficulty in breathing in any of the yoga postures. If you do, back out of the posture and do not go so deep into them. Listen to your body.

The rejuvenating yoga flow sequence will take approximately 75 minutes to complete.

Rejuvenating Yoga Flow Sequence Chart

Beginner's Sun Salutation Sequence (Repeat 3 times)

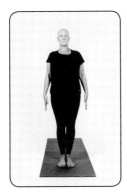
Tadasana

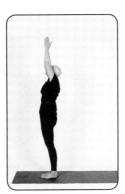
ONE

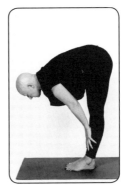
TWO

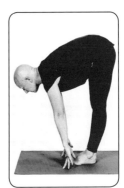
THREE

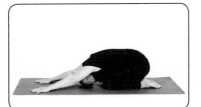
FOUR

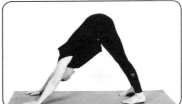
FIVE

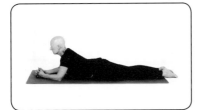
SIX (Hold for 5 breaths)

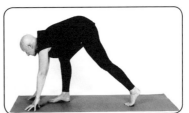
SEVEN

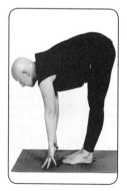

EIGHT

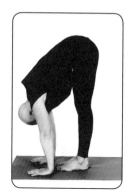

NINE

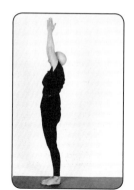

TEN

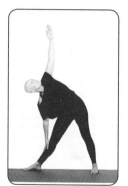

Triangle pose

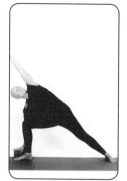

Extended side angle

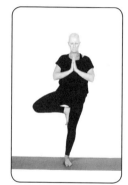

Tree pose

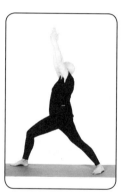

Warrior 1

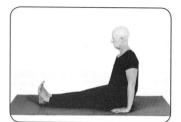

Staff pose

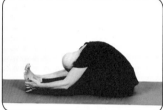

Seated forward bend

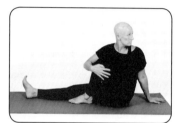

Seated twist

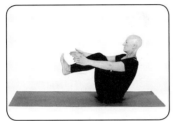

Boat posture

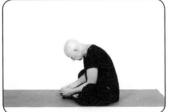

Cobbler pose

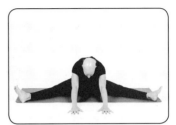

Seated wide angle pose

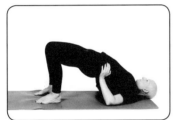

Supported back bend

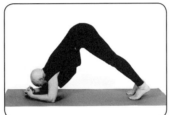

Dolphin posture

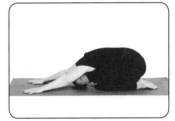

Child's pose

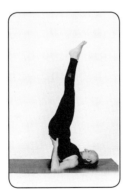

Shoulder stand

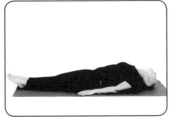

Fish pose

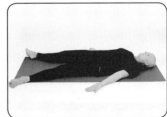

Savasana

Beginner's Sun Salutation Sequence

a. Standing with both feet together, lift and engage your thigh muscles. Suck your stomach in, towards your chest, keeping both shoulders and hands relaxed in Tadasana (mountain pose).

b. One – inhale both hands to the sky, tilt head backwards and gaze towards your hands.

c. Two – exhale fold forwards with flat back. Rest both hands onto the shin or floor and gaze towards your nose.

d. Three – inhale and look up, gaze towards your nose.

e. Four – exhale, walk back and go into child's pose.

f. Five – inhale, going into sphinx posture.

g. Six – exhale into downward-facing dog. Imagine this as an inverted V-shape. Legs hip-width apart, hands shoulder-width apart. Straighten your arms and press your palms firmly onto the floor. Straighten your legs and work on bringing the back of your heels onto the floor. You can bend your knees if your hamstrings are very tight. Try to evenly distribute your weight between the front and back of your body.

h. *Drishiti* – gaze towards your navel. Stay here for five breaths. Breathe deeply.

i. Seven – inhale, look up and walk both feet forwards.

j. Eight – exhale forward, and fold into a forward bend.

k. Nine – inhale and come back to standing tall with a straight spine. Palms together and gaze towards your hands.

l. Ten – exhale and release both hands to the side. Round 1 completed.

m. Repeat two more rounds of sun salutation. Take it at your own pace, and if any point fatigue sets in, just come down and rest in child's pose.

n. You can work towards building strength and stamina by repeating three rounds of sun salutations.

> **Comments:** The sun salutation is a dynamic sequence, designed to be aerobic and get the heart rate increases to help benefit patients. It is not uncommon for beginners to feel out of breadth or dizzy going through the sequence, or to experience their hands/shoulders feeling tired whilst holding downward-facing dogs. With sufficient practice, this will become easier as your body develops further strength and stamina during the recovery process.

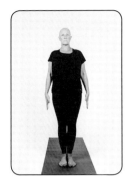

Tadasana

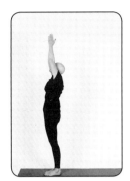

ONE

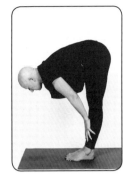

TWO

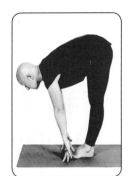

THREE

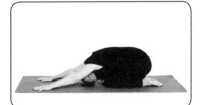

FOUR

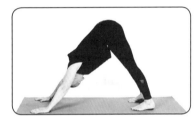

FIVE

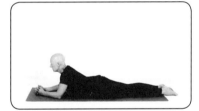

SIX (Hold for 5 breaths)

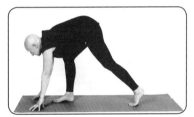

SEVEN

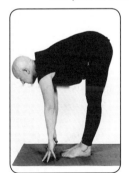

EIGHT

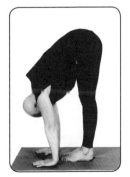

NINE

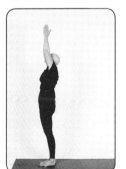

TEN

Triangle Pose

a. Inhale and step your right feet out three feet apart. Turn your left foot at 45 degrees with your right foot pointing forwards

b. Exhale open both arms to shoulder-height apart and reach your right hand forward, resting your right on your thigh (A), just below your knee (B), or your shin (C), keeping both legs straight and strong.

c. Inhale and rotate your body to the sky. Straighten your left hand and gaze towards your left hand.

d. *Hastagrai drishiti* – gaze towards your left hand.

e. Stay here and breathe deeply for five breaths.

f. Inhale and come all the way back up.

g. Exhale, turning your right foot at 45 degrees and putting your left foot forward, coming all the way down your left side and again, choosing your appropriate edge.

h. Inhale and rotate your body to the sky. Straighten your right hand and gaze towards your left hand.

i. *Hastagrai drishiti* – gaze towards your right hand.

j. Stay here and breathe deeply for five breaths.

k. Inhale and come all the way back up.

l. Exhale, and bring both feet in front of the mat, standing upright in mountain posture.

Comments: The triangle pose is a great posture to engage core muscles and it encourages lateral stretches along the back and opening of the chest. If you feel discomfort in the neck, you can also gaze at the front of the front foot. Try to evenly distribute the weight on both feet and press the balls of the feet firmly into the floor, keeping the back foot grounded, creating a strong firm foundation.

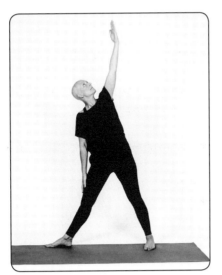

A

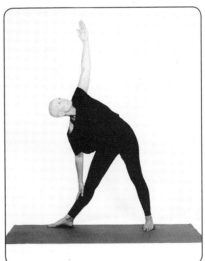

B

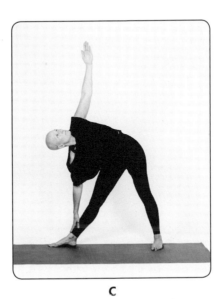

C

Extended Side Angle Pose

a. Inhale; step your right feet out 4-5 feet wide apart and turn your left foot at 45 degrees.
b. Exhale, bending your right knee towards 90 degrees. Ensure your right heels are in line with your right knees.
c. Inhale; place your right elbow/forearm near the top of your knee without sinking your entire body weight (A). Place the block vertically (B) or horizontally for support, if required (C).
d. Exhale; straighten your arms out to 45 degrees and *hastagrai drishiti* – gaze towards your left hand.
e. Breathe deeply for five breaths.
f. On your last inhale, straighten your front leg and come all the way to standing gently.
g. Exhale, turn to the other side and repeat the extended side angle pose on the right side, holding the *hastagrai drishiti* gaze towards your left hand.
h. Remain here for another five deep breaths.
i. Come out of the posture by straightening the left leg and come all the way to standing, feet together at the front of the mat.

Comments: There is a tendency in this posture to collapse the front body. Try to root the back foot firmly into the floor and distribute the weight of the body evenly between the two feet. The extended side stretch also helps to loosen the intercostal muscles between the ribcage, helping to expand your breath.

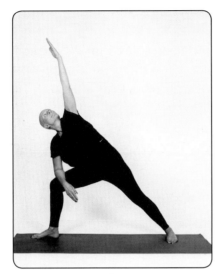

A

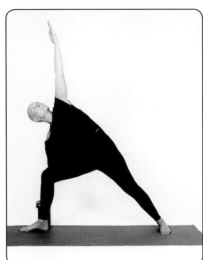

B

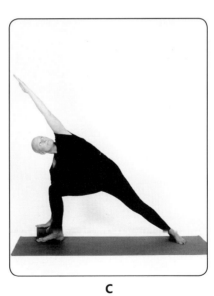

C

Tree Pose

a. From standing, keeping your shoulders relaxed and spine straight, engage your core muscles by tucking your stomach in and lift it towards your chest. Root both feet firmly onto the floor and feel your gluteal muscles engage.

b. Inhale, and bring your left hand onto your left waist.

c. Exhale, and keeping your left leg strong and straight, shift the weight of the body to the left slightly.

d. Inhale, placing your right foot against your inner thigh and bring both hands into a prayer position and raise both hands to the sky – hands shoulder-width apart (A). If this is not possible, place your right foot underneath your knee joint (B) or above your ankle (C).

e. Keeping your core strong, point your tailbone towards to floor. There is a tendency to overarch your lower back in this posture.

f. *Drishti* – gaze towards a fixed point on the floor in front of you to help balance.

g. Inhale and exhale deeply for five breaths.

h. Exhale, releasing your hands and right foot onto the floor.

i. Repeat on the left side.

Comments: There is a tendency for practitioners to over-arch their lower back in this posture. Remember to tuck the tailbone in and engage your core muscles to stabilise yourself. You may also find your legs shaking or a strong burning sensation in your glut muscles. With time, you will feel more stable in this posture as your muscles grow stronger.

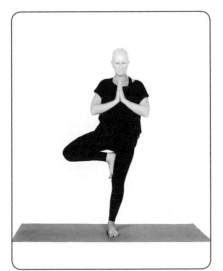

A

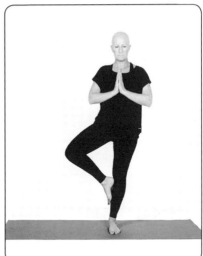

B

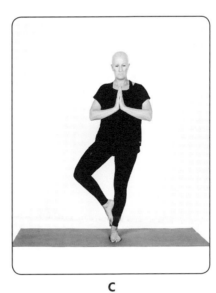

C

Warrior 1

a. Inhale and step your right feet three feet apart, turning your left foot in at a 45-degree ankle, with your right foot straight, parallel to the mat.

b. Inhale, square your hips and bend your right knee towards 90 degrees – knee in line with heel. Bring both hands up towards the sky, palms together, and tilt your head back slightly, gazing towards your hands (A). You can also have your hands apart, parallel to the shoulder, if there is too much strain on your shoulders.

c. *Hastagrai drishiti* – gazing towards your hands.

d. Stay here for five deep breaths.

e. Inhale and straighten your front leg, keeping your hands raised and where they are, turning your body towards the back now. Your right foot should be at 45 degrees, with your left foot pointing forwards.

f. Exhale, squaring your hips and sink your left knee towards 90 degrees. Check your knees are in line with your heels again. Bring both hands up towards the sky, palms together, and tilt your head back slightly, gazing towards your hands (A). You can also have your hands apart, parallel to the shoulder, or elbows bent, if there is too much strain on your shoulders.

g. Stay here for five deep breaths.

h. Inhale, straightening you right leg, coming all the way back to standing.

Comments: It is important to remember to keep the knee directly above the heel of the front foot to prevent potential injuries that could result from overstraining your knee joints. Engage the back foot strongly and root the outer edge of the back foot firmly into the floor.

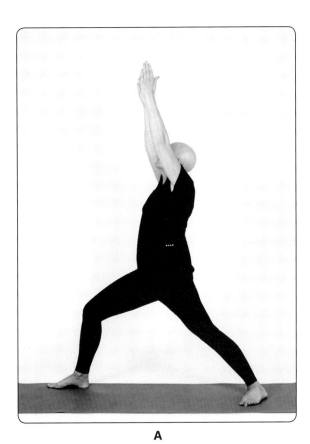

A

"There is a Zen story about a man riding a horse that is galloping very quickly. Another man, standing alongside the road, yells at him, "Where are you going?" and the man on the horse yells back, "I don't know. Ask the horse." I think that is our situation. We are riding many horses that we cannot control."
- Venerable Thich Nhat Hanh, Being Peace

Staff Pose

a. From standing, come down to sitting with both legs straight in front of you.

b. Inhaling, press both hands, aligned with your hips, onto the floor, palms flat (A). If you experience tightness in your lower back and find it hard to keep your spine straight, and also, if you experience tightness in your hamstrings, which is preventing you from straightening your legs, bend your knees (B) and put some folded blankets for additional support, if required (C).

c. Exhale, chin down. Keeping your legs active, engage your quadriceps, keeping your spine tall and arms straight.

d. *Nasagrai drishti* – gaze towards the top of the nose and stay here for five breaths.

e. Inhale, chin up and relax your shoulders.

Comments: This pose might look deceptively passive and simple at first glance. But in reality, there are several opposing forces at work in this posture, which make it quite challenging, whilst encouraging the building of core strength. For example, the sit-bones and heels move away from each other. The sacrum sinks down while the spine is lengthened. The chest opens and lifts, whilst the hands are firmly pressed down into the floor.

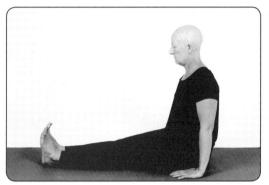

A

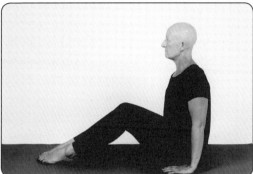

B

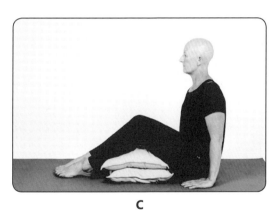

C

Seated Forward Bend

a. Staying in the staff pose, inhale and bring both hands up to the sky. Keep your spine straight and your shoulders relaxed.

b. Exhale, keeping both arms straight, your spine straight, and forward bend, reaching as far as your hands can reach, and wrapping both hands outside of your feet (A), or rest your hands on your shin (B). If you have your knees bent, you can rest your forehead on your knees (C)/(D).

c. *Padhayoragrai drishti* – gaze towards your toes. Keep your shoulders relaxed.

d. Breathing deeply here, hold for 10 breaths.

e. On your last inhale, come back up to a straight spine.

f. Exhale, coming back to the staff pose, and rest both hands on the floor next to your waist.

Comments: If you feel discomfort or pain in your lower back, bend your knees and come out of the posture slowly. You should also keep your spine long and shoulders relaxed in the posture. Do not pull yourself into the forward bend as it will only serve to tighten the shoulders more. There is also a tendency for the outer edge of the feet to roll inwards; point your toes back and keep the feet actively engaged, which will help to lengthen and stretch the hamstring further.

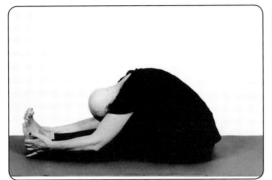

A

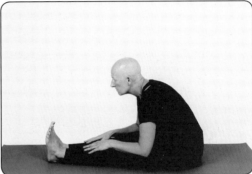

B

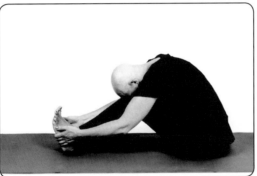

C

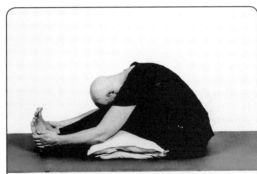

D

Seated Twist

a. From a staff pose, inhale and bend the right leg and place your heel near the sit-bone. Place your right hand on the floor behind you.

b. Exhale, twist and rotate from the lower spine and hold the right knee with your left hand (A). If you have had surgery, you might experience discomfort or pain along the chest/shoulder area and you should move your right feet forward to ease off the intensity of the pose (B).

c. Inhale, lengthen your spine, and turn your gaze over the right shoulder.

d. *Parsva drishti* – gaze towards the back.

e. Stay here for five deep breaths.

f. Inhale, keeping your spine straight, and rotate and turn your body to the front.

g. Exhale, release your hands and straighten both legs.

h. Inhale, placing your left hand on the floor behind you.

i. Exhale, twist and rotate from the lower spine. Hold the left knee with your right hand and select your appropriate edge (C/D).

j. Inhale and bend the left leg and place your heel near the sitbone. Place your left hand on the floor behind you.

k. *Parsva drishti* – gaze towards the back.

l. Stay here for another five deep breaths.

m. Inhale, keeping your spine straight, and rotate and turn your body to the front.

n. Exhale, release your hands and straighten both legs.

Comments: This posture is particular helpful for those who have undergone reconstructive surgery. It helps to release the tension around the head/neck and shoulder region, whilst also encouraging healing of scar tissues. Furthermore, it stretches and loosens the spine, toning and conditioning the nerves along the spinal cord. It can also help to relieve neck pain and mild forms of sciatica. If you find that your lower back hunches too much in this posture and it is preventing you from twisting to the side, sit on a yoga block to add some height and help straighten the spine.

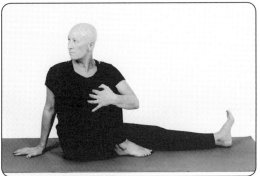

A

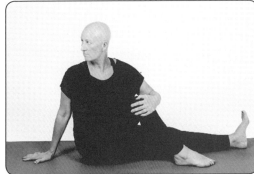

B

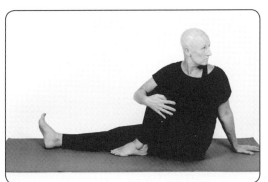

C

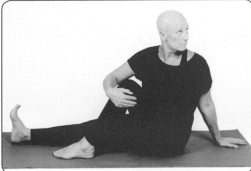

D

Boat Posture

a. Inhale, bringing both knees into the chest and wrap both hands underneath your knees for support. Keep your back straight and your core muscle engaged.

b. Exhale and straighten both legs out parallel to the floor (A). Release both hands to the side, palms facing in, and hold the posture for five breaths (B). If this is too difficult, you can remain in option A or try to support your lower back with a brick (C).

c. *Padhayoragrai drishiti* – gaze towards your toes

d. Exhale, releasing both feet onto the floor and resting your hands onto the floor.

e. Rest here for five breaths and then repeat the boat posture four more times.

f. Come into a simple seated, cross-legged posture.

Comments: The greatest challenge in this posture is to keep the lower back straight and lifted away from the floor. For those who have undergone any surgical procedures around the abdominal area, it would be advisable to take this slowly and allow your core strength to rebuild in a sustainable manner. Listen to your body and stay in option A.

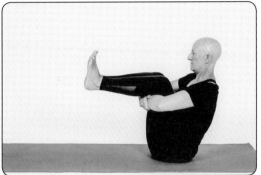

A

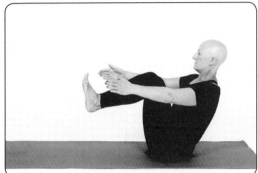

B

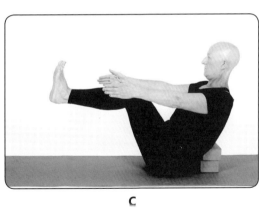

C

Cobbler Pose

a. From a simple seated, cross-legged posture, exhale, drawing both feet into the groin and grab the top of the feet with both hands (A). You may also sit on a yoga brick if you find it difficult sitting cross-legged (B).
b. Inhale and lift your spine and chin, gazing directly in front of you.
c. Exhale, keeping the chin tucked in and the spine straight. Tilt forward with your pelvis and lean as far forward as you can.
d. *Nasagrai drishiti* – gaze at the top of the nose.
e. Hold here for five breaths.
f. Inhale, keeping your spine long, and sit up gently.
g. Exhale, release the feet and straighten both legs.

Comments: Whilst tilting your pelvis forward, you may feel pressure against the groin and lower abdominal area. If you find this posture too intense, stay in option A or B. By opening the feet, you will still reap the benefit of the gentle hip opening that results from this posture.

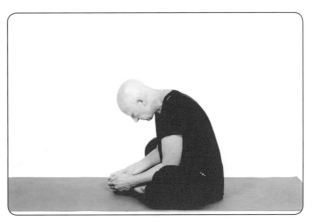

A

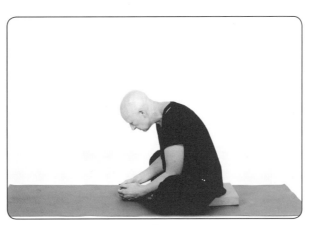

B

Seated Wide Angle Pose

a. Exhale and bring both legs far apart (A). You may also want to sit on a yoga brick in this posture if you find your lower back rounding excessively.

b. Inhale and lift your spine and chin, gazing directly in front of you.

c. Exhale, maintaining length in your spine. Tilt forward with your pelvis as far as you are comfortable (B).

d. *Nasagrai drishiti* – gaze at the top of the nose.

e. Hold here for five breaths.

f. Inhale as you sit up gently.

g. Exhale, bend your knees and bring both knees together to come out of the posture. Straighten both legs in front of you.

Comments: Whilst tilting forward, it is important to keep pointing the knees towards the sky and do not roll them in toward the floor. If you find this posture too intense, stay at your appropriate edge.

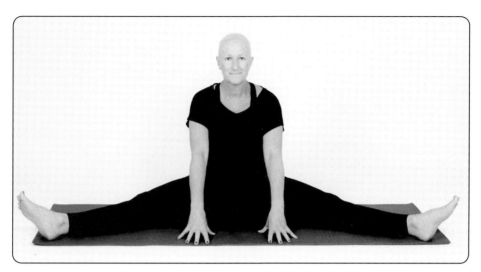

A

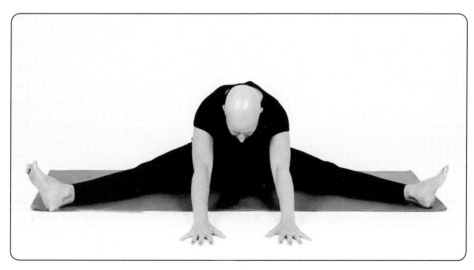

B

Supported Back Bend

a. Exhale and come to lie back onto the floor.
b. Inhale, bend your knees and bring them close towards your buttocks (A).
c. Exhale and press your elbows onto the floor
d. Inhale, arch your back, lift your chest and support both hips with your hands as you come into a supported back bend (B), and hold here for 10 breaths. Keep your core strong.
e. *Nasagrai drishti* – gaze at the top of the nose.
f. On your last exhale, gently lower your spine back onto the floor, keeping your knees bent.
g. Inhale, bringing both knees into your chest (C).
h. Gently rock sideways to release the tension on your back.

Comments: If you feel a sharp pain or severe discomfort in your neck or lower back then release the posture and reset with greater muscular support. Keep both legs parallel to each other, engage the quadriceps and lift your hips towards the sky whilst pressing the feet firmly into the floor. Engage your core muscle and drop your shoulders back, opening your chest. Feel the front stretch on your body – there shouldn't be undue pressure on the lower back. If you have had mastectomy or breast reconstruction surgeries, you may want to modify and stay at your appropriate edge whilst opening the chest.

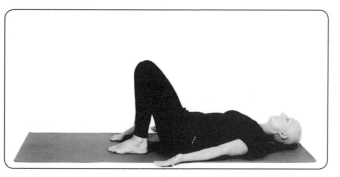

A

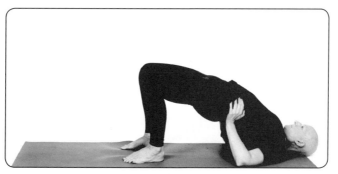

B

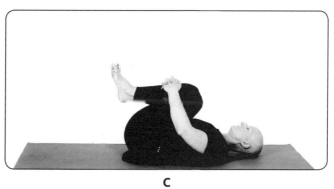

C

Child's Pose

a. Transition from lying back on the floor and come into a kneeling position. Bring knees and feet together and sit on the back of your soles.

b. Exhale, reach forwards with your fingers and rest your forehead onto the floor. Keep both hands straight in front of you and relax completely onto the floor.

c. *Nasagrai drishti* – gaze towards your nose and breathe deeply for 20 breaths.

d. Using your arms for support, gently push yourself to an upright position.

Comments: The child's pose is a very healing posture and stretches the spine. The gentle compression of the stomach and chest encourages circulation and promotes healing in those areas of the body.

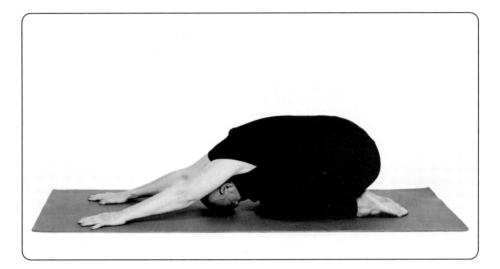

"We do so much, we run so quickly, the situation is difficult, and many people say, "Don't just sit there, do something." But doing more things may make the situation worse. So you should say, "Don't just do something, sit there." Sit there, stop, be yourself first, and begin from there."
– Venerable Thich Nhat Hanh, Being Peace

Dolphin Posture

a. Inhale from kneeling position and place your forearms on the floor with your shoulders directly above your wrists. Firmly press your palms together and your forearms into the floor.

b. Curl your toes under, then exhale and lift your knees away from the floor. At first keep the knees slightly bent and the heels lifted away from the floor. Lengthen your tailbone away from the back of your pelvis and press it lightly toward the pubis. Against this resistance, lift the sitting bones toward the ceiling, and from your inner ankles draw the inner legs up into the groins.

c. Continue to press the forearms actively into the floor. Firm your shoulder blades against your back, then widen them away from the spine and draw them toward the tailbone. Hold your head between the upper arms; don't let it hang or press heavily against the floor.

d. You can straighten both legs to stretch out your hamstrings (A), but if your upper back rounds it's best to keep them bent (B). Continue to lengthen your tailbone away from the pelvis and lift the top of your sternum away from the floor.

e. Stay between 30 seconds to one minute. Then release your knees to the floor with an exhale.

Comments: The dolphin pose is a very challenging pose and is the foundation of building sufficient core and upper body strength for more advanced postures like headstands. If this is too intense for you, you can choose to stay in the child's pose.

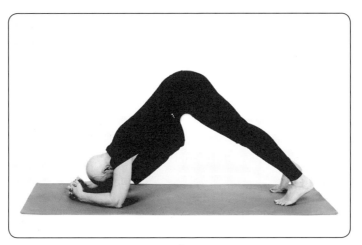

A

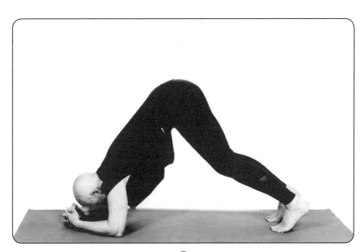

B

Shoulder Stand

a. Transitioning from the child's pose/dolphin pose, lie flat on the floor.

b. Exhale and roll up onto your shoulders, supporting the back with both hands and placing both hands close to the spine.

c. Inhale, bend both knees towards the chest and gently lift both legs towards the sky in a perpendicular position (A).

d. If this is too difficult or places too much pressure on your neck, you can leave your hips on the floor and bring your legs to the sky (B), or adopt the supported shoulder stand posture with the wall as your support (C).

e. *Nasagrai drishti* – gazing towards your nose.

f. Remain here for 25 breaths.

g. Exhale and come all the way down slowly to lie flat on the floor.

Comments: If you feel discomfort or a sharp pain in the neck, back off and come out of the posture completely. The bulk of the weight should be distributed evenly across the shoulders, upper arms and elbows. You can still reap the benefits of the inversion without coming to the full posture. Potential benefits include decreasing varicose veins, reducing the heart rate and regulating hormone production, massaging the thyroid gland and strengthening of the immune system.

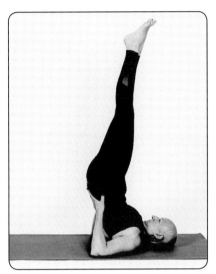

A

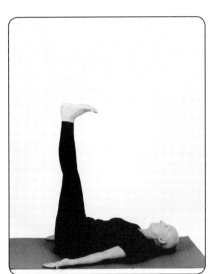

B

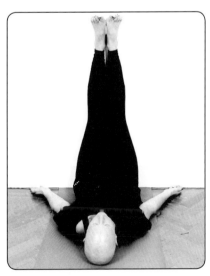

C

Fish Pose

a. Exhale and bring your hands close to your sides with your palms flat on the floor.

b. Inhale, gently arching your back and bringing the crown of your head onto the floor, opening your throat and releasing the tension around your shoulders. This is a counter-posture to the shoulder stand and releases residual tension around the upper back area (A). You may also wish to place a pillow or cushion behind your upper back for additional support (B). Alternatively, for a stronger upper back/throat opening, place a yoga block horizontally along the upper back, in between the shoulder blades (C).

c. *Nasagrai drishti* – gazing towards your nose.

d. Hold here for five breaths.

e. Exhale, coming all the way down to the floor.

Comments: The fish pose is the counter posture to the shoulder stand and help release tension around the shoulders. By lifting the chin and drawing the head backwards, it helps to increase blood flow to the throat area, stimulating the thyroid gland. The thyroid gland is about two-inches long and lies in front of your throat below the Adam's apple. It produces Triiodothyronine (T3) and Thyroxine (T4) hormones, which are important in regulating many bodily functions.

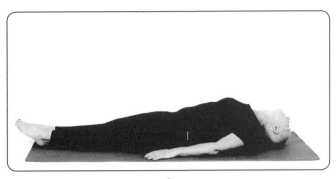

A

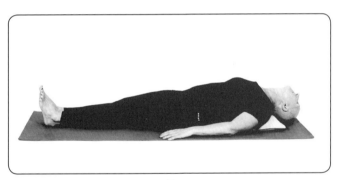

B

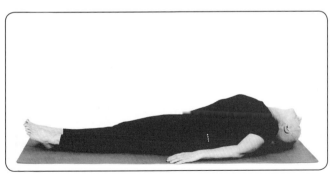

C

Final Relaxation – Savasana

a. Inhale, bring your hands away from your waist and open your palms up, facing the sky.
b. Exhale and close your eyes.
c. Breathe normally here and totally relax your body. Release any unwanted tension you may have.
d. Stay here for 10 – 15 minutes and let your body absorb the impact of your practice.

Comments: Some of the potential benefits of *Savasana* include relieving mild depression, fatigue, headaches, high blood pressure and insomnia. Sometimes, *Savasana* is also said to be the hardest yoga pose as one may find it very difficult to stay awake and remain focused whilst lying down on the floor. *Savasana* helps us learn how to completely surrender, quieten the internal chatter, and make room for inner peace and harmony.

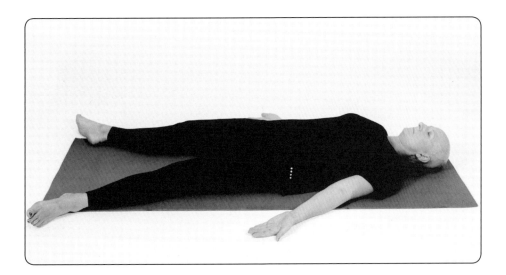

'Yoga is the journey of the self, through the self, to the self"
– The Bhagavad Gita

Dynamic Yoga Flow Sequence

The dynamic yoga flow sequence is specifically designed for cancer survivors who have worked through both the healing and rejuvenating sequences during their recovery journey.

If you are ready for a more dynamic, stronger practice – this sequence is for you.

You should never experience pain in your bones/joints or difficulty in breathing in any of the yoga postures. If you do, back out of the posture and do not go so deep into them. Listen to your body.

The dynamic yoga flow sequence will take approximately 90 minutes to complete.

Sun Salutation Sequence (Repeat 5 times)

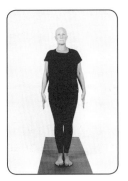

Tadasana

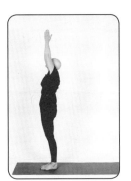

ONE

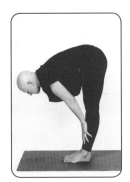

TWO

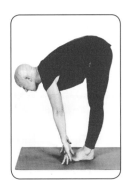

THREE

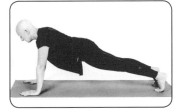

FOUR (A)

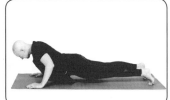

FOUR (B)

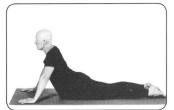

FIVE

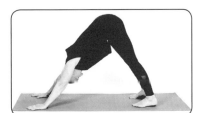

SIX (Hold for 5 breaths)

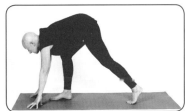

SEVEN

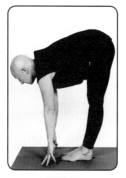

EIGHT

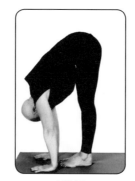

NINE

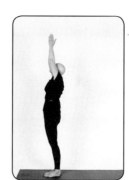

TEN

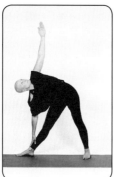

Triangle pose

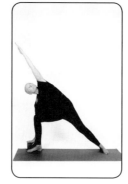

Extended side angle

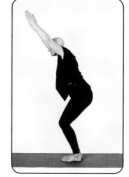

Chair pose

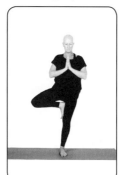

Tree pose

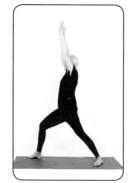

Warrior 1

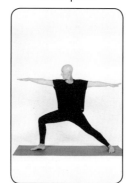

Warrior 2

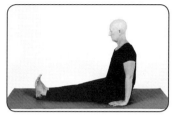

Staff pose

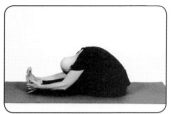

Seated forward bend

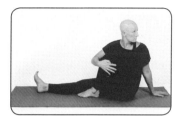

Seated twist

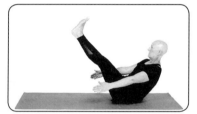

Boat posture

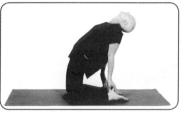

Camel pose

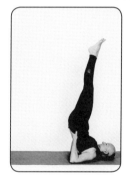

Shoulder stand

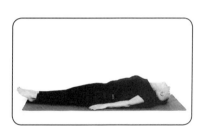

Fish pose

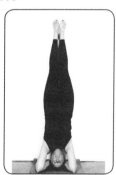

Headstand

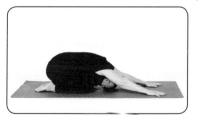

Child's pose

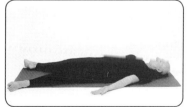

Savasana

Sun Salutation Sequence

a. Standing with both feet together, lift and engage your thigh muscles. Suck your stomach in and lift it towards your chest, keeping both shoulders relaxed.

b. One – inhale both hands to the sky, tilt your head backwards and gaze towards your hands.

c. Two – exhale and fold forwards with a flat back. Rest both hands onto the shin or floor and gaze towards your nose.

d. Three – inhale, look up and gaze towards your nose.

e. Four a – exhale and jump back into the plank position.
   Four b – bending your elbow 90 degrees for a push-up position.

f. Five – inhale, going into upward-facing dog, with your chest open and your arms straight.

g. Six – exhale into downward-facing dog. Imagine this as an inverted V-shape with your legs hip-width apart and your hands shoulder-width apart. Straighten your arms and press your palms firmly onto the floor. Straighten your legs and work on bringing the back of your heels onto the floor. You can bend your knees if your hamstrings are very tight. Try to evenly distribute your weight between the front and back of your body. *Nabi chakra drishti* – gaze towards your navel. Stay here for five breaths. Breathe deeply.

h. Seven – inhale, look up and walk or jump both feet forwards.

i. Eight – exhale and forward fold into a forward bend.

j. Nine – inhale and come back to standing tall with a straight spine. Put your palms together and gaze towards your hands.

k. Ten – exhale and release both hands to your sides. Round 1 completed.

l. Repeat two more rounds of sun salutation. Take it at your own pace, and if at any point fatigue sets in, just come down and rest in the child's pose.

m. You can work towards building strength and stamina by repeating five rounds of sun salutations.

Comments: The Sun salutation A sequence is a more advanced version of the previous beginner's sun salutation sequence, requiring a greater arm strength and flexibility to move through the sequence. With practice, the synchronisation of breath and movement will be an energising, uplifting experience that will serve as the "warm up" of your practice.

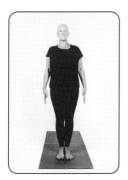

Tadasana

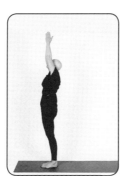

ONE

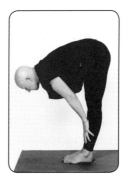

TWO

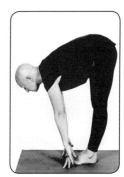

THREE

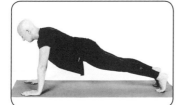

FOUR (A)

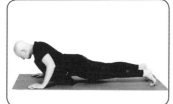

FOUR (B)

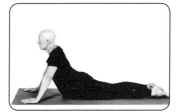

FIVE

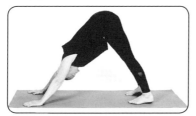

SIX (Hold for 5 breaths)

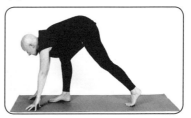

SEVEN

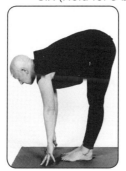

EIGHT

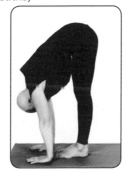

NINE

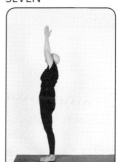

TEN

Triangle Pose

a. Inhale and step your feet out, three feet apart. Turn your left foot at 45 degrees and your right foot pointing forwards.

b. Exhale, open both arms apart at shoulder-height and reach your right hand forward, resting it on your thighs (A), below your right knee (B) or on your right shin (C). Keep both legs straight and strong.

c. Inhale and rotate your body to the sky, straighten your left hand and gaze towards your left hand.

d. *Hastagrai drishiti* – gaze towards your left hand.

e. Stay here and breathe deeply for five breaths.

f. Inhale and come all the way back up.

g. Exhale, turning your right foot at 45 degrees and your left foot forward. Coming all the way down you're your left side and again, choosing your appropriate edge, rest your right hand just below your knee (A), grabbing your right shin (B) or touching your right big toe (C). Keep both legs straight and strong.

h. Inhale and rotate your body to the sky, straighten your left hand and gaze towards your right hand.

i. *Hastagrai drishiti* – gaze towards your right hand.

j. Stay here and breathe deeply for five breaths.

k. Inhale and come all the way back up.

l. Exhale and bring both feet in front of the mat, standing upright in a mountain pose.

Comments: The triangle pose is a great posture to engage core muscles and encourage lateral stretches along the back and opening of the chest. If you feel discomfort in the neck, you can also gaze at the front of the front foot. Try to evenly distribute the weight on both feet and press the balls of the feet firmly into the floor, keeping the back foot grounded, creating a strong firm foundation.

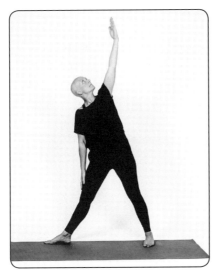

A

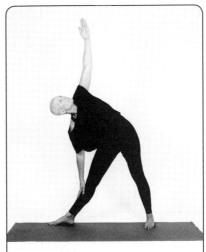

B

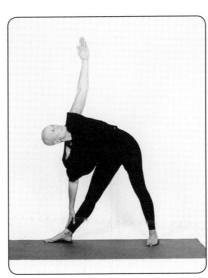

C

Extended Side Angle Pose

a. Inhale, step your feet out 4-5 feet apart, and turn your left foot at 45 degrees.
b. Exhale, bending your right knee at a 90-degree angle. Ensure your right heel is in line with your right knee.
c. Inhale and place your right elbow/forearm near the top of your knee without sinking your entire body weight (A). Place the block vertically (B) or horizontally for support if required (C).
d. Exhale, straighten your arms out at 45 degrees and *hastagrai drishiti* – gaze towards your left hand.
e. Breathe deeply for five breaths.
f. On your last inhale, straighten your front leg and come all the way to standing gently.
g. Exhale, turn to the other side and repeat the extended side angle pose on the left side, holding a hastagrai drishiti gaze towards your RIGHT hand.
h. Remain here for another five deep breaths.
i. Come out of the posture by straightening the left leg and come all the way to standing, feet together, at the front of the mat.

Comments: There is a tendency in this posture to collapse the front body. Try to root the back foot firmly into the floor and distribute the weight of the body evenly between the two feet. The extended side stretch also helps to loosen the intercostal muscles between the ribcage, helping to expand your breath.

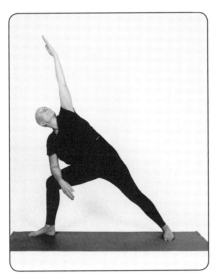

A

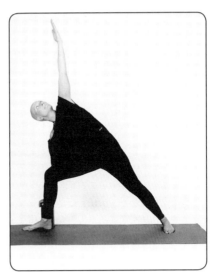

B

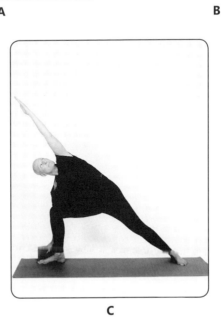

C

Tree Pose

a. From standing, keeping your shoulders relaxed and spine straight, engage your core muscles by tucking your stomach in and lift it towards your chest. Root both feet firmly onto the floor and feel your gluteal muscles engage.

b. Inhale and bring your left hand onto your left waist.

c. Exhale, keeping left leg strong and straight, and shift the weight of the body to the left slightly.

d. Inhale, placing your right foot against your inner thigh and bring your hand into a prayer position – hands shoulder-width apart (A). If this is not possible, place your right foot underneath your knee joint (B) or above your ankle (C).

e. Keeping your core strong, point your tailbone towards to floor. There is a tendency to overarch your lower back in this posture.

f. *Drishti* – gaze towards a fixed point on the floor in front of you to help balance.

g. Inhale and exhale deeply for five breaths.

h. Exhale, releasing your hands and right foot onto the floor.

i. Repeat on the left side.

Comments: There is a tendency for practitioners to over-arch their lower back in this posture. Remember to tuck the tailbone in and engage your core muscles to stabilise yourself. You may also find your legs shaking or a strong burning sensation in your glut muscles. With time, you will feel more stable in this posture as your muscles grow stronger.

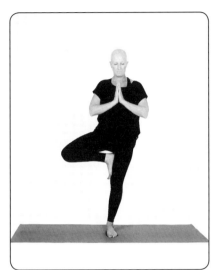

A

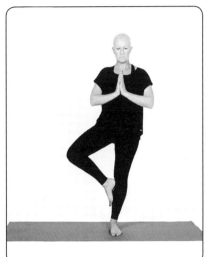

B

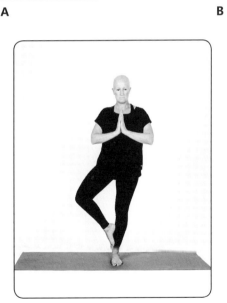

C

Chair Pose

a. Stand with your feet and knees together.
b. Inhale and drop your hips towards the floor as far as you can go. Imagine sitting on an imaginary chair and fold forwards, bringing both hands towards the sky (A). You can sink deeper towards 90 degrees if you want to further challenge and tone your thigh muscles (B).
c. Exhale, lengthening the spine and look up, palms together, gazing towards your hands.
d. *Hastagrai drishiti* – gaze towards your hands or directly in front of you if your shoulder muscles are tight.
e. Hold here and take five deep breaths.
f. Inhale, straighten both legs and come back up to a standing mountain posture.

Comments: Remember to keep the knees, ankles and toes touching in this posture. Press the feet firmly into the floor and tilt the weight slightly towards the heel. Feel the opposing forces of gravity pulling you towards the floor, whilst your hands point towards the sky, creating an equal, dynamic, opposing stretch. You may also feel a burning sensation in your thigh muscles. That is good – it is working to keep you supported. Go to your appropriate edge.

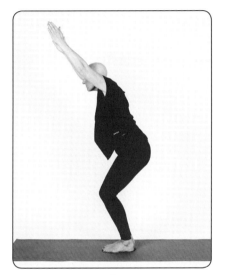

A

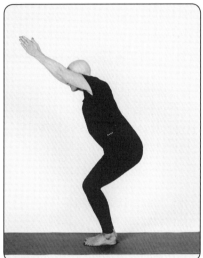

B

> **"Anywhere we go, we will have our self with us;**
> **we cannot escape ourselves."**
> – Venerable Thich Nhat Hanh

Warrior 1

a. Inhale and step your feet three feet apart, turning your left foot at 45 degrees and your right foot parallel to the mat.

b. Exhale and place both hands onto your hips, squaring your hips as much as possible.

c. Inhale, bending your right knee – keep your knee in line with your heel. Bring both hands up towards the sky, palms together, and tilt your head back slightly, gazing towards your hands (A). For a stronger pose, you can bend your knee towards 90 degrees (B).

d. *Hastagrai drishiti* – gazing towards your hands.

e. Stay here for five deep breaths.

f. Inhale and straighten your front leg, keeping your hands raised and where they are, turning your body towards the back now. Put your right foot at 45 degrees and your left foot pointing forwards.

g. Exhale, squaring your hips, and sink your left knee towards 90 degrees. Check that your knees are in line with your heels again. Bring both hands up towards the sky, palms together, and tilt your head back slightly, gazing towards your hands (A). You can also have your hands apart, parallel to the shoulder (B), or elbows slightly bent if there is too much strain on your shoulders (C).

h. Stay here for five deep breaths

i. Inhale, straightening you front leg and coming all the way back to standing.

Comments: It is important to remember to keep the knee directly above the heel of the front foot to prevent potential injuries that could result from overstraining your knee joints. Engage the back foot strongly and root the outer edge of the back foot firmly into the floor.

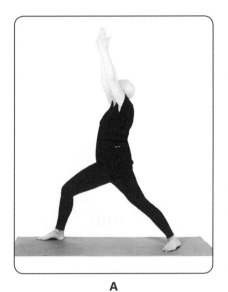

A

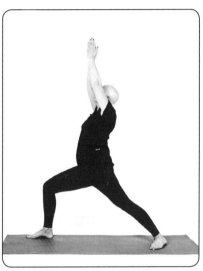

B

"Yoga does not remove us from the reality or responsibilities of everyday life but rather places our feet firmly and resolutely in the practical ground of experience. We don't transcend our lives; we return to the life we left behind in the hopes of something better."

– Donna Farhi

Warrior 2

a. Inhale and step your feet five feet apart, turning your left foot at 45 degrees and your right foot parallel to the mat.
b. Exhale, bending your right knee and ensure that heel is in front of knee (A).
c. Inhale, open your arms parallel to the floor and, rotating your head sideways. Adopt the *Angustha Ma Dyai drishiti* – gaze towards your thumbs and stay here for five deep breaths. For a challenge, lower your knees towards 90 degrees by bringing your knee in line with your heel (B).
d. Stay here for five deep breaths.
e. Inhale and straighten your front leg, keeping your hands parallel to the floor and turning your body towards the back now. Put your right foot at 45 degrees and your left foot pointing forwards
f. Exhale, sinking your left knee towards 90 degrees. Check that your knees are in line with your heels again.
g. Stay here for five deep breaths.
h. Inhale, straightening your left leg, coming all the way back.
i. Exhale and come to sit in a seated staff posture.

Comments: There is a tendency to over-arch your lower point in this posture, creating undue strain on it. Engage your core muscle and point the tailbone towards the floor. You might also feel an intense stretch in your inner groin. Press firmly on both feet, equally distributing the weight between the front and the back foot to stabilise the body, maintain grace and equilibrium in the posture.

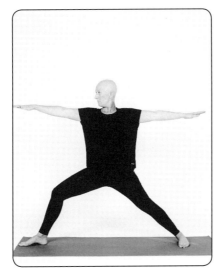

A

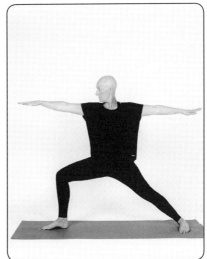

B

"The only journey is the journey within."
– Rainer Maria Rilke, Bohemian-Austrian poet and novelist

Staff Pose

a. From standing, come down to sitting with both legs straight in front you.
b. Inhaling, press both hands aligned with your hips onto the floor, palms flat.
c. Exhale, chin down, keeping your legs active and engaging your quadriceps. Keep your spine tall and your arms straight.
d. *Nasagrai drishti* – gaze towards the top of the nose and stay here for 10 breaths.
e. Inhale, chin up and relax your shoulders.

Comments: This pose might look deceptively passive and simple at first glance. But in reality, there are several opposing forces at work in this posture, which make it quite challenging, whilst encouraging the building of core strength. For example, the sit-bones and heels move away from each other. The sacrum sinks down whilst the spine is lengthened. The chest opens and lift whilst the hands are firmly pressed down into the floor.

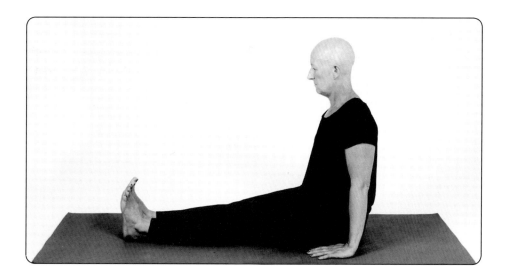

'Yoga teaches us to cure what need not be endured and
endure what cannot be cured"
– B.K.S Iyengar

Seated Forward Bend

a. Staying in the staff pose, inhale and bring both hands up to the sky. Keep your spine straight and your shoulders relaxed.
b. Exhale, keep both arms straight, your spine straight, and forward bend, reaching as far as your hands can. Wrap both hands outside of your feet (A) or rest your hands on your thighs (B).
c. *Padhayoragrai drishti* – gaze towards your toes. Keep your shoulders relaxed.
d   Breathing deeply here, hold for 10 breaths.
e. On your last inhale, come back up WITH a straight spine.
f. Exhale, coming back to a staff pose and rest both hands on the floor next to your waist.

Comments: If you feel discomfort or pain in your lower back, bend your knees and come out of the posture slowly. You should also keep your spine long and shoulders relaxed in the posture. Do not pull yourself into the forward bend as it will only serve to tighten the shoulders more. There is also a tendency for the outer edge of the feet to roll inwards. Point your toes back and keep the feet actively engaged, which will help to lengthen and stretch the hamstring further.

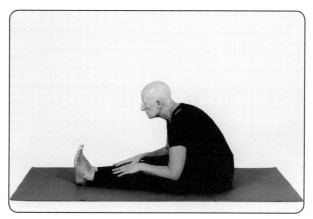

A

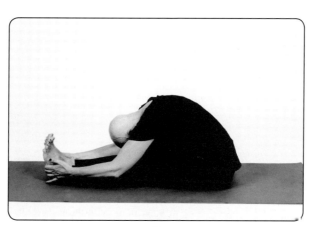

B

Seated Twist

a. From a staff pose, inhale and bend the right leg and place your heel near the sit-bone. Place your right hand on the floor behind you.

b. Exhale, twist and rotate from the lower spine and hold the right knee with your left hand (A). If you have had surgery, you might experience discomfort or pain along the chest/shoulder area and you should move your right feet forward to ease off the intensity of the pose (B).

c. Inhale, lengthen your spine and turn your gaze over the right shoulder.

d. *Parsva drishti* – gaze towards the back.

e. Stay here for five deep breaths.

f. Inhale, keeping your spine straight, and rotate and turn your body to the front.

g. Exhale, release your hands and straighten both legs.

h. Inhale and place your left hand on floor behind you.

i. Exhale, twist and rotate from the lower spine. Hold the left knee with your right hand and select your appropriate edge (C/D).

j. Inhale, lengthen your spine and turn your gaze over the left shoulder.

k. *Parsva drishti* – gaze towards the back.

l. Stay here for another five deep breaths.

m. Inhale, keeping your spine straight, rotate and turn your body to the front.

n. Exhale, release your hands and straighten both legs.

Comments: This posture is particular helpful for those who have undergone reconstruction surgery. It helps to release the tension around the head/neck and shoulder region, whilst also encouraging the healing of scar tissues. Furthermore, it stretches and loosens the spine, toning and conditioning the nerves along the spinal cord. It can also help to relieve neck pain and mild forms of sciatica. If you find that your lower back hunches too much in this posture and it is preventing you from twisting to the side, sit on a yoga block to add some height and help straighten the spine.

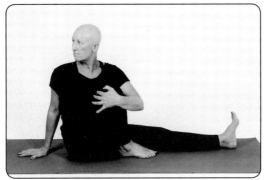

A

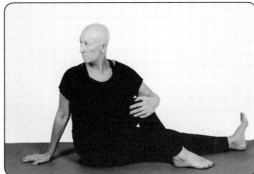

B

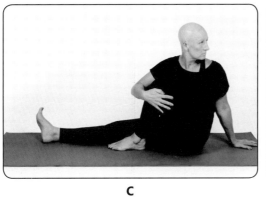

C

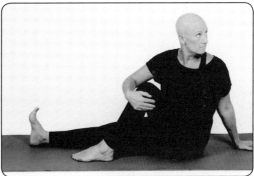

D

Boat Posture

a. Inhale, bringing both knees into your chest and wrap both hands underneath your knees for support. Keep your back straight and your core muscle engaged.

b. Exhale and straighten both legs out, parallel to the floor. Release both hands to the side, palms facing in, and hold the posture for five breaths (A). You can also straighten both legs (B).

c. *Padhayoragrai drishiti* – gaze towards your toes.

d. Exhale, releasing both feet onto the floor and resting your hands on the floor.

e. Rest here for five breaths and then repeat the boat posture four more times.

f. Come into a simple seated, cross-legged posture.

Comments: The greatest challenge in this posture is to keep the lower back straight and lifted away from the floor. For those who have undergone any surgical procedures around the abdominal area, it would be advisable to take this slowly and allow your core strength to rebuild in a sustainable manner. Listen to your body and stay in option A.

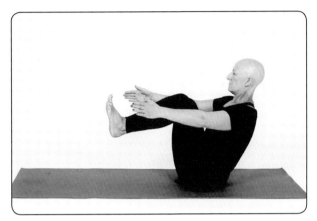

A

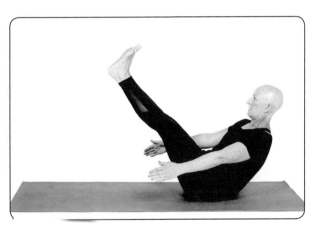

B

Camel Posture

a. Inhale and come forward into a kneeling position.
b. Exhale and bring both hands onto your waist.
c. Inhale and lift your chest with your core muscle engaged (A). You can use folded blankets for additional cushioning and support of your knees.
d. Exhale and slowly drop back as far as you can go, without putting undue strain on your lower back (B)
e. You can either stay here or choose to bring your hands onto the top of your heels (C), opening your chest and throat.
f. *Urdhva drishiti* – gaze upwards/up to the sky.
g. Hold here for five breaths. Breathe deeply.
h. To exit the posture, inhale and sit on the heels, placing your hands on the floor.

Comments: The camel posture is an intense back bend that arches the sacral/lumbar spine, stretches the hip flexors and opens the shoulders. If you feel dizzy, do not drop the head too far back. If your back muscle starts to spasm, back out of the posture and do the gentler versions.

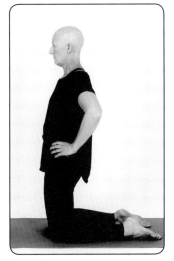

A

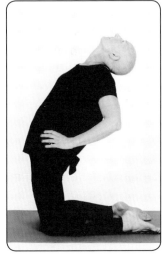

B

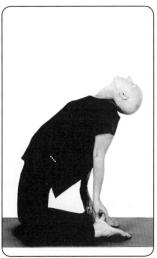

C

'It is good to tame the mind, which is difficult to hold in and flighty, rushing wherever it listeth; a tamed mind brings happiness"
– Sacred texts of The Dhammapada, The Buddha

Shoulder Stand

a. Transition from the camel pose and come to lie flat on the floor.
b. Exhale and roll up onto your shoulders, supporting the back with both hands, placing both hands close to the spine.
c. Inhale and bend both knees towards the chest, gently lifting both legs towards the sky into a perpendicular position.
d. *Nasagrai drishti* – gazing towards your nose.
e. Remain here for 25 breaths.
f. Exhale and come all the way down slowly to lie flat on the floor.

Comments: If you feel discomfort or sharp pain in the neck, back off and come out of the posture completely. The bulk of the weight should be distributed evenly across the shoulders, upper arms and elbows. You can still reap the benefits of the inversion without coming to the full posture. Potential benefits include decreasing varicose veins, reducing your heart rate and regulating hormone production, massaging the thyroid glands and strengthening of the immune system.

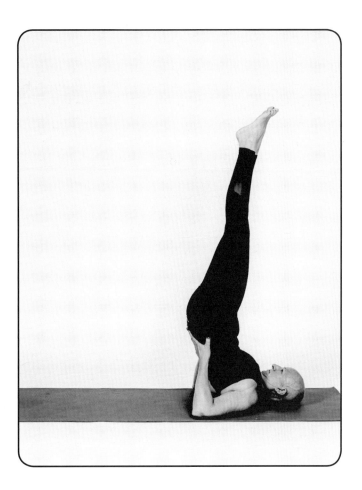

"Better it is to live one day wise and meditative than to live
a hundred years foolish and uncontrolled"
– Sacred texts of The Dhammapada, The Buddha

Fish Pose

a. Exhale and bring your hands close to your sides, palms flat on the floor.
b. Inhale, gently arching your back, and bring the crown of your head onto the floor, opening your throat and releasing the tension around your shoulders. This is a counter-posture to the shoulder stand and releases residual tension around the upper back area.
c. *Nasagrai drishti* – gazing towards your nose.
d. Hold here for five breaths.
e. Exhale, coming all the way down to the floor.

Comments: The fish pose is the counter posture to the shoulder stand and help releases tension around the shoulders. By lifting the chin and drawing the head backwards, it helps to increase blood flow to the throat area, stimulating the thyroid gland. The thyroid gland is about two-inches long and lies in front of your throat below the Adam's apple. It produces Triiodothyronine (T3) and Thyroxine (T4) hormones, which are important in regulating many bodily functions.

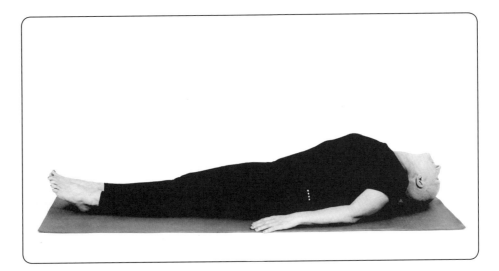

"99% practice, 1% theory."
– Guruji K. Pattahbi Jois, Founder of the Ashtanga Yoga Research
Institute Mysore, India

Headstand

a. Coming into the child's pose from the fish pose, you can use the wall for support to attempt the headstand at the beginning phase.
b. Inhale, and place your elbows on the floor, shoulder-width apart. Interlock the fingers to form a triangular base.
c. Exhale and place the crown of your head on the floor between the hands for support (A).
d. Inhale, straighten both legs and come into <u>a forearm</u> downward-facing dog (B).
e. Exhale, engage your core by tucking your stomach in, walk your legs towards the chest and gently bend both knees into a half headstand, keeping your spine straight and strong (C).
f. Keep pointing your toes and do not collapse your lower back, keeping your ribs tucked in. You may use the wall for support and prevent yourself from falling over (D). Alternatively, you may also ask for assistance from a yoga instructor to support you during your headstand practice (E).
g. Stay here for 20 breaths.
h. On your last exhale, start by bending your knees and gently bringing both feet to the floor.

Comments: Remember to keep the neck straight in the pose and the majority of the weight should be distributed on the elbows and arms and not the head. If you feel discomfort or pain in the neck or head, back out of the posture immediately. It is also common for practitioners to feel fear whilst attempting headstands. B. K. S. Iyengar once said, "The best way to overcome fear is to face with equanimity the situation of which one is afraid." With regular practice, you can begin to reap the benefits as the headstand is also known as the King of Asanas, and you will gain mental clarity as you encourage blood flow towards the head whilst it relaxes the heart muscles as de-oxygenated blood flows more easily from the extremities back to the heart.

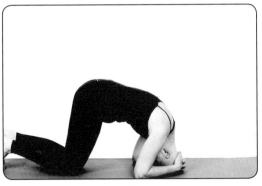

A

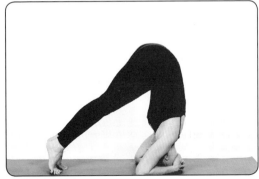

B

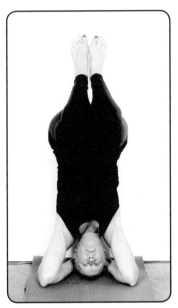

C

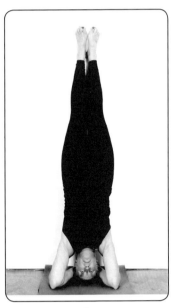

D

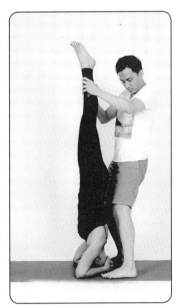

E

Child's Pose

a. Transition from a headstand; inhale and come into a kneeling position on the floor, bring knees and feet together and sit on the back of your soles.

b. Exhale, reach forwards with your fingers and rest your forehead onto the floor. Keep both hands straight in front of you and relax completely onto the floor (A). If you head doesn't reach the floor, you can use a bolster for support.

c. *Nasagrai drishti* – gazing towards your nose and breathe deeply for 5 breaths.

d. Using your arms for support, gently push yourself to an upright position.

Comments: The child's pose is a very healing posture and stretches the spine. The gentle compression of the stomach and chest encourages circulation and promotes healing in those areas of the body.

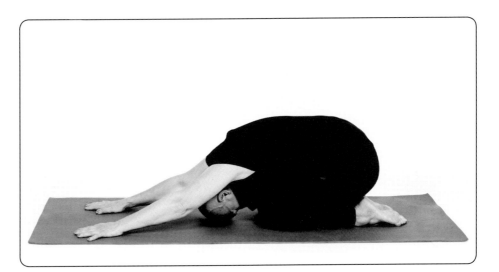

"Yoga is the cessation of the fluctuation of the mind."
– Patañjali

Final relaxation – Savasana

a. From a seated position, inhale and bring your legs out slightly wider than hip-width apart
b. Exhale, and with the support of your elbows, come to lie down on your back.
c. Inhale, bring your hands away from your waist and open your palms up, facing the sky.
d. Exhale and close your eyes.
e. Breathe normally here and totally relax your body. Release any unwanted tension you may have.
f. Stay here for 10 – 15 minutes and let your body absorb the impact of your practice

Comments: Some of the potential benefits of *Savasana* include relieving mild depression, fatigue, headaches, high blood pressure and insomnia. Sometimes, *Savasana* is also said to be the hardest yoga pose, as one may find it very difficult to stay awake and remain focused whilst lying down on the floor. *Savasana* helps us learn how to completely surrender, quieten the internal chatter and make room for inner peace and harmony.

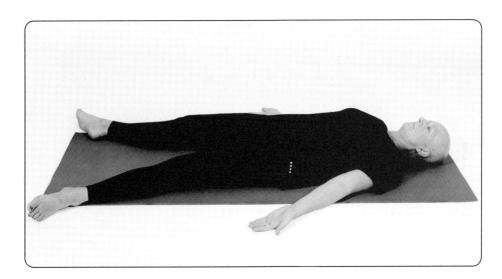

"Meditation is to be aware of what is going on: in your body, in your feelings, in your mind, and in the world."
– Venerable Thich Nhat Hanh, Being Peace

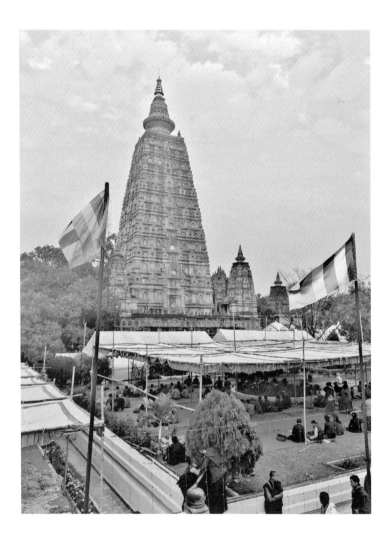

"Feelings come and go like clouds in a windy sky.
Conscious breathing is my anchor."
– Venerable Thich Nhat Hanh

Pranayama

The Sanskrit word *Pranayama* is made up of two words – *prana* (life force or vital energy) and *ayama* (expansion or extension). *Pranayama* literally translates as "the expansion of vital energy", and this form of yoga breathing exercises can be considered as a form of mindfulness breathing, which requires the practitioner to be conscious of their own breathing habits and make the necessary adjustments to allow the body to rejuvenate and maximise its energy level by nourishing the body organs through our breath.

On average, we breathe 12 – 18 times per minute [23], 21,600 times a day. Breathing allows the oxidation of glucose to generate energy in the form of Adenosine triphosphate (ATP), required to sustain physiological functions. Most of us, preoccupied with our daily activities or thoughts, are not conscious in the way we breathe. As a result, a majority of us breathe in a shallow way, utilising only a small part of our lung capacity. In addition, stress/tension, bad posture and restrictive clothing can also lead to shallow and/or rapid breathing. *Pranayama* practice aims to promote a slow, rhythmic and deep breathing, which helps the practitioner create a sense of calm and peace, promoting mental wellbeing in the process.

Pranayama can be practiced anytime, right before or after the recovery yoga sequences, or as a standalone practice. The following tips that might enhance your experience of a *pranayama* practice are as follows:

1) Take a nice, long, warm bath.
2) Wear loose clothing.
3) Practice on an empty stomach.
4) Choose a clean, quiet and well-ventilated place.
5) Breathe through your nose, unless otherwise specified.

Level 1 – Single nostril breathing

1) Sit in a comfortable, cross-legged position or sit with a cushion or use the wall as support.
2) Gently close your eyes and place your left hand onto your left knee.
3) Ensure your spine is straight, your chest is open and your shoulders are relaxed.
4) Tuck your chin inwards, slightly towards the throat.
5) Bring your right hand into *nasikagra mudra* by folding the index and middle finger into the palm of the hand. *Mudra* is a Sanskrit word that means gesture or attitude, which in yoga philosophy is believed to help the practitioner develop a more refined consciousness by manipulating the flow of *prana*.
6) Bring your right hand to the right side of your nose and close the right nostril with your right thumb (A).
7) Inhale for four seconds through the left nostril.
8) Exhale for eight seconds through the left nostril.
9) Repeat this five times.
10) Close the left nostril with your pinkie finger (B).
11) Inhale for four seconds through the right nostril.
12) Exhale for eight seconds through the right nostril.
13) Bring your right hand onto your right knee.
14) Breath normally through both nostrils for five regular breaths.
15) Gently open your eyes and enjoy the peace and stillness.
16) Repeat five or more rounds of single nostril breathing to gain the full benefit.

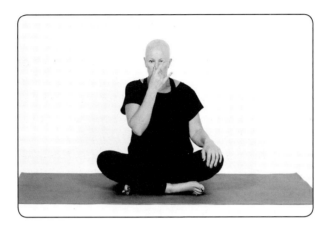

A

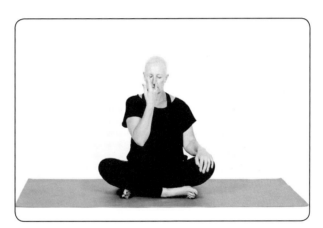

B

"Peace comes from within. Do not seek it without."
– The Buddha, Enlightened One

Level 2 – Alternate nostril breathing without breath retention

1) Sit in a comfortable, cross-legged position or sit with a cushion or use the wall as support.
2) Gently close your eyes and place your left hand onto your left knee.
3) Ensure your spine is straight, your chest is open and your shoulders are relaxed.
4) Tuck your chin inwards, slightly towards the throat.
5) Bring your right hand into *nasikagra mudra* by folding the index and middle finger into the palm of the hand. *Mudra* is a Sanskrit word that means gesture or attitude, which in yoga philosophy is believed to help the practitioner develop a more refined consciousness by manipulating the flow of *prana*.
6) Bring your right hand to the right side of your nose and close the right nostril with your right thumb.
7) Inhale for four seconds through the left nostril.
8) Close the left nostril with your pinkie finger.
9) Exhale for eight seconds through the right nostril.
10) Inhale for four breaths through the right nostril.
11) Bring your left hand to the left side of your nose and close the left nostril with your left thumb.
12) Exhale for eight seconds through the left nostril.
13) This completes one full round of the breath.
14) Repeat this for five or more rounds to gain the full benefit.
15) Breath normally through both nostrils for 20 regular breaths to close your practice.

Level 3 – Alternate nostril breathing with full breath retention

1) Sit in a comfortable, cross-legged position or sit with a cushion or use the wall as support.
2) Gently close your eyes and place your left hand onto your left knee.
3) Ensure your spine is straight, your chest is open and your shoulders are relaxed.
4) Tuck your chin inwards, slightly towards the throat.
5) Bring your right hand into *nasikagra mudra* by folding the index and middle finger into the palm of the hand. *Mudra* is a Sanskrit word that means gesture or attitude, which in yoga philosophy is believed to help the practitioner develop a more refined consciousness by manipulating the flow of *prana*.
6) Bring your right hand to the right side of your nose and close the right nostril with your right thumb.
7) Inhale for four seconds through the left nostril.
8) Hold your breath for four seconds.
9) Close the left nostril with your pinkie finger.
10) Exhale for four seconds through the right nostril.
11) Inhale for four breaths through the right nostril.
12) Hold your breath for four seconds.
13) Bring your right thumb to the right side of your nose close the left nostril with your left thumb.
14) Exhale for eight seconds through the left nostril.
15) This completes one full round of the breath.
16) Repeat this for five or more rounds to gain the full benefit.
17) Breath normally through both nostrils for 30 regular breaths to close your practice.

Further Reading

Following a complete recovery, you may wish to explore and experiment with the different schools of yoga tradition to deepen your understanding and practice of yoga. I have listed a range and summary of the most common yoga traditions.

Ashtanga yoga is a physically demanding form of yoga, founded by Pattabhi Jois in the early 1900s for young, adolescent males with physical strength and untamed minds [24]. In a typical practice, it consists of a set routine sequence of *asanas* (postures), which begins with sun salutations, followed by the standing sequence, primary - intermediate - advanced series, and finally, the closing sequence. Also, a key part of practice that differentiates this type of yoga from the other forms is the practice of *vinyasa*, which essentially is series of lifting and jumping push ups when transitioning between postures, creating excess heat to remove ama (toxins), which makes this suitable for those looking for an aerobic, physical strenuous workout.

Anusara yoga is a modern school of hatha yoga, founded by John Friend in 1997 [25]. Friend derives this school of yoga from Iyengar but re-incorporates elements of Hindu spirituality in it. A typical lesson involves an opening "lecture" by the instructor, which discusses yoga and aspects of Hindu philosophy, followed by short chanting, and then with a sequence of postures that focus on the alignment of energies, in particular, "heart opening" postures. Lessons close with chanting. It is suitable for people interested in the philosophy behind yoga and perhaps those wanting to experiment and adventure the newer schools of yoga.

Hatha yoga is a system of yoga introduced by Yogi Swatmarama, a yogic sage in the 15th century in India [26]. It can be considered an all-round form of yoga routine – it focuses on all the different aspects of yoga without placing too much emphasis on just postures. It encourages the building of physical strength and stamina via sun salutations, meditative practice, and also encourages development of concentration. Sometimes, teachers give discourses/stories of how to bring yoga out of the classroom/yoga mat into everyday living. It is generally regarded as a gentle form of yoga, suitable for beginners and all levels alike.

Insight yoga is what I would call a "middle path" yoga [27], inspired by Buddhist philosophies of incorporating both yang and yin asanas in the practice, with classes typically finishing off with extended periods of meditation to encourage the development of inner awareness. Sarah Powers, a well-respected insight yoga master, discusses meditation, and emphasises that yoga is only a tool/stepping stone in helping yogis to attain proficiency in meditation and does not treat yoga as a pure physical exercise regime.

Iyengar yoga is created by B. K. S. Iyengar, and is a form of Hatha yoga, known for its use of props, such as belts, blocks, and blankets, as aids in performing postures. The props enable students to perform the postures correctly, minimising the risk of injury or strain, and making the postures accessible to both young and old. The development of strength, mobility, and stability are emphasised through the postures [28]. The practice can be considered static and focuses a lot on correct alignment, core strength and flexibility. Postures are typically held for 10 – 20 minutes each. It is also considered as a complementary yoga form to Ashtanga yoga, and Iyengar is great for those recovering from injuries, great for beginners to master asanas, and those wanting to focus on flexibility.

Jivamukti yoga is derived from the Sanskrit word *jivanmuktih*, wherein *jiva* is the individual living being, and *mukti* is the liberation of an individual from the Buddhist/ Hindu belief of the cycle of death and rebirth. Jivamukti classes are generally 90 minutes in length [29]. Each class focuses on a theme, based on a globally-set "focus of the month", which is explored through "dharma talks", Sanskrit chanting, reflections on the modern relevance of yoga scripture, music, asanas, pranayama and meditation. The largest portion of the class consists of vinyasa, where the teacher guides the practitioner through a vigorous sequence of poses that is synchronised with steady breathing. Poses include inversions, such as headstand and shoulder stand. During the vinyasa phase, the teacher assists practitioners with hands-on adjustments. The class concludes with a period of deep relaxation and meditation.

Power yoga is founded by Larry Schultz, an early student of Jois, who is often regarded as the pioneer of power yoga that is popularised in the West [30]. It might sometimes be referred to as "Rocket yoga" as well. This form of yoga, as the name suggests, is extremely physically demanding, with heavy emphasis on the more vigorous asanas and the warrior sequences throughout the practice.

Sivananda yoga is a non-proprietary form of Hatha yoga, derived following the teachings of Swami Sivananda [31]. This form of yoga is considered gentle and the emphasis is on full yogic breathing, coupled with series of basic sequences – pranayama and frequent relaxation is involved. Chanting is often involved through the class as well and in between postures. It is suitable for beginners and those looking for de-stress, mental relaxation, and to learn more about yogic breathing techniques.

Yin yoga was founded by Master Paulie Zink, who taught Paul Grilley. Its primary focus is on passive asanas that stimulate the parasympathetic nervous systems and connective joint tissues, which are involved in the unconscious regulation of internal organs – "rest and digest" activities. The yin yoga class consists of a routine 26 passive postures, which are held for as long as possible – usually 5 – 30 minutes each [32]. The teachings of Paul Grilley incorporate ideas related to traditional Chinese medicine and Qigong. Yin yoga can be incredibly restorative and is suitable for those seeking a completely restorative class, especially when you have not much physical energy but are still wanting a way to de-stress and do yoga at the end of day.

References

[1]   R. A. Weinberg, "The Hallmarks of Cancer", *Cell*, vol. 100, no. 1, pp. 57-70, 2000.

[2]   Patanjali, The Yoga Sutras of Patanjali; The Book of the Spiritual Man, RareBooksClub.com, 2012.

[3]   P. CL, "How does yoga reduce stress? A systematic review of mechanisms of change and guide to future inquiry", *Health Psychol Rev*, vol. Sep 9(3), pp. 379-96, 2015.

[4]   M. Kjær, "Effect of adrenaline on glucose kinetics during exercise in adrenalectomised humans", *The Journal of Physiology*, vol. Sep 15; 519(Pt 3), p. 911-921, 1999 .

[5]   H. AC, "Exercise and circulating cortisol levels: the intensity threshold effect", *J Endocrinol Invest*, vol. Jul; 31(7), pp. 587-91, 2008.

[6]   A. Matthews, Yoga Anatomy - 2nd Edition, Human Kinetics Publishers, 2011.

[7]   S. American, "Why does lactic acid build up in muscles? And why does it cause soreness?", 23 Jan 2006. [Online]. Available: http://www.scientificamerican.com/article/why-does-lactic-acid-buil/.

[8]   S. P, "Immediate effect of yogic visual concentration on cognitive performance", *J Tradit Complement Med*, vol. 6(1), pp. 34-6, 2015.

[9]   M. E, "Yoga and Cognition: A Meta-Analysis of Chronic and Acute Effects", *Psychosom Med*, vol. 77(7), pp. 784-97, 2015.

[10] D. Higgins, "Men, don't let your ego dictate your exercise routine", 10 Nov 2010. [Online]. Available: http://www.standard.co.uk/lifestyle/health/men-dont-let-your-ego-dictate-your-exercise-routine-6534444.html.

[11] P. E. Wändell, "Increased heart rate variability but no effect on blood pressure from 8 weeks of hatha yoga – a pilot study", *BMC Res Notes*, vol. 6:59, 2013.

[12] P. A. McCullough, "Potential Adverse Cardiovascular Effects From Excessive Endurance Exercise", *Mayo Clin Proc*, vol. 87(6), p. 587-595, 2012.

[13] CRUK, "CRUK - Yoga", [Online]. Available: http://www.cancerresearchuk.org/about-cancer/cancers-in-general/treatment/complementary-alternative/therapies/yoga.

[14] L. Cohen, "Randomized, controlled trial of yoga in women with breast cancer undergoing radiotherapy", *J Clin Oncol*, vol. 32(10), pp. 1058-65, 2014.

[15] K. G. JK, "Yoga's impact on inflammation, mood, and fatigue in breast cancer survivors: a randomized controlled trial", *J Clin Oncol*, vol. 32(10):, pp. 1040-9, 2014.

[16] B. JE, "Yoga reduces inflammatory signaling in fatigued breast cancer survivors: a randomized controlled trial" *Psychoneuroendocrinology*, vol. 43, pp. 20-9, 2014.

[17] S. F, "Yoga for Patients with Early Breast Cancer and its Impact on Quality of Life – a Randomized Controlled Trial", *Geburtshilfe Frauenheilkd*, vol. 73 (4), pp. 311-317, 2013.

[18] B. J. AM, "Yoga Intervention for Patients With Prostate Cancer Undergoing External Beam Radiation Therapy: A Pilot Feasibility Study", *Integr Cancer Ther*, vol. pii: 1534735415617022, 2015.

[19] F. JM, "A pilot study of the feasibility and outcomes of yoga for lung cancer survivors", *Oncol Nurs Forum. 2014 Mar* , vol. 41(2), pp. 162-74, 2014.

[20] F. A, "Lymphedema after breast or gynecological cancer: use and effectiveness of mainstream and complementary therapies", *J Altern Complement Med*, vol. 17(9), pp. 867-9, 2011.

[21] D. SC, "Restorative yoga for women with ovarian or breast cancer: findings from a pilot study", *J Soc Integr Oncol*, vol. Spring; 6(2), pp. 47-58, 2008.

[22] M. KM, "Multicenter, randomized controlled trial of yoga for sleep quality among cancer survivors", *J Clin Oncol*, vol. 31(26), pp. 3233-41, 2013.

[23] K. E. Barrett, Ganong's Review of Medical Physiology, 24th Edition (Lange Basic Science), McGraw-Hill Medical, 2012.

[24] P. Jois. [Online]. Available: http://kpjayi.org/the-practice.

[25] A. Y. S. Community, "Anusara Yoga Shri Community". [Online]. Available: http://www.anusara.com/.

[26] Y. Swatmarama, "Yogi Swatmarama autobiography". [Online]. Available: http://en.wikipedia.org/wiki/Yogi_Swatmarama.

[27] S. Powers, "Insight yoga". [Online]. Available: http://www.sarahpowers.com/approach.html.

[28] U. Iyengar Yoga Institute, "Iyengar Yoga Institute, UK". [Online]. Available: http://www.iyi.org.uk/.

[29] J. Y. London, "Jivamukti Yoga London". [Online]. Available: http://www.jivamuktiyoga.co.uk/.

[30] L. Schulz, "Larry Schulz autobiography". [Online]. Available: http://en.wikipedia.org/wiki/Larry_Schultz.

[31] I. S. Organization, "International Sivananda Organization". [Online]. Available: http://www.sivananda.org/.

[32] P. Grilley, "Yin Yoga". [Online]. Available: http://www.yinyoga.com/index.php.

Further Resources

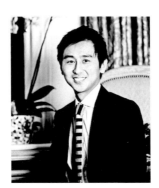

Dr Yoga – www.dryoga.co.uk

Dr Yoga ® was founded by Dr Jimmy Kwok in 2011 to promote the benefits that yoga could bring for cancer patients and recovering survivors. Jimmy gained his MA in Natural Sciences from Emmanuel College, University of Cambridge and his doctorate degree in Clinical Oncology (Breast Cancer) at Imperial College, London. Jimmy has also interned at Harvard Medical School, Boston USA and the Oncology Department at Great Ormond Street Hospital, London. He is also a registered Yoga Alliance UK RYT200 yoga instructor and has developed extensive experience in promoting and teaching yoga classes at Maggie's Cancer Centre, West London, within the Charing Cross Hospital Campus.

Having worked in the oncology field for over a decade, he has recognised that the psychological, emotional and physical support for cancer patients is often overlooked, and has developed a series of materials in supporting the recovery for cancer patients and survivors.

Visit Dr Yoga's website at **www.dryoga.co.uk** for further information.

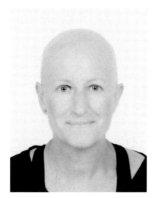

ABC Diagnosis - www.abcdiagnosis.co.uk

Jo had primary breast cancer in 2007 when Jo was 38 with a 5-month old daughter and 2.5 year old son. A full mastectomy and reconstruction, chemotherapy, radiotherapy, Herceptin and other treatments. A year on Jo was diagnosed with secondary breast cancer. Jo is now treated every 3 weeks that are keeping the cancer in check. 2 years on Jo has had a radical sternotomy to reduce the cancer load as her disease is mainly confined to just two areas of the bones currently.

Jo created a website that launched in 2013 where she blogs about her experiences and the various projects she is involved with to do with breast cancer as a patient advocate. The website is dedicated to supporting primary and secondary breast cancer patients make informed choices with information and up to date news on treatments, breast surgeries, consultants, hospital and useful links.

By participating in modelling for this book, she hopes that the thoughtful sequences put together by Dr Kwok will benefit others affected by breast cancer.

Here is a link to her full story at http://www.abcdiagnosis.co.uk/about-abcd/my-story/.

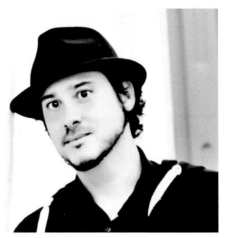

Scott Ralph Studio – www.ScottRalphstudio.com

Scott was born in New York City to Swedish and Italian parents. He became a world traveller at a very young age, thanks to his parents, due to their busy lives and his father's international business ventures.

Having lived part time in several countries, his family moved permanently to London when he was 12. He attended Millfield School then spent a year abroad in Moscow, Russia. Throughout his life, he has always kept his innate love of exploring the world, including its different cultures and languages, which reflects a lot in his photographic work. Scott is also fluent in four languages.

After finishing university in London, and having spent all his life to this point learning and studying, Scott was finally ready to spread his wings and go solo. For the past nine years, Scott has been successfully photographing for a very varied client base worldwide, and his main goal at the moment is working on his stunning coffee table books, whilst doing shoots where and when he can in London and throughout the UK.

These include a book on Africa, a high fashion book, which incorporates important aspects of life and several equality issues, which he feels very strongly about, a book on his recent expedition to the Antarctic, and a trilogy of world travel with a twist, set to be sponsored by a famous sunglasses company.

Scott had an immediate interest in doing this book when he was asked to be involved. In part, due to his close friendship with the book's author, Dr Jimmy Kwok, but also as Scott's mother, who has been a huge influence in his life, has been an avid fan of daily yoga for the past 15 years, and maintains to this day that it saved her life and changed her body and mind for the better in so many ways. Scott's father sadly passed away in 2007 after a long battle with prostate cancer, so any causes that help spread awareness and help people overcome this unjust illness that affects so many people is very personally close to his heart.

Scott sees his future one day going back to his roots and, using good old-fashioned film and a dark room, creating "one of a kind works of art". While he is well travelled and an extremely accomplished photographer, Scott absorbs the world around him and all that it has to offer, and is therefore still learning and growing every day.

"Photography is truth and fantasy. It is the art of loving and feeling what you do. The camera in this is irrelevant; it is having the true ability to photograph the beauty in what you see. When you photograph your passions in life, you see very clearly."

Index

A

B

C